First Aid Yourself

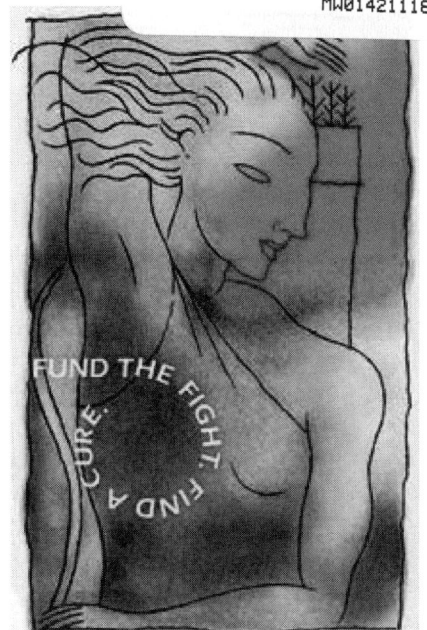

Essential Breast Cancer Websites

OAKWOOD ARTS AND SCIENCES EDITION

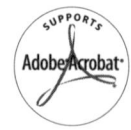

Don't Miss the eBook

First Aid Yourself, Essential Breast Cancer Websites
is also published as an "eBook" and your purchase
of this premium edition entitles you to download
the free Electronic Edition in Adobe Software's PDF Format.
The Electronic Edition is identical in appearance to the
Printed Edition you now hold in your hands, but all
Internet hyperlinks are active—a simple click
will take you to the Website mentioned.
In addition, the Table of Contents, Subject Index and
complete Appendix of Websites are also hyperlinked.

For download instructions, please register your copy of
First Aid Yourself, Essential Breast Cancer Websites
at:
http://www.firstaidyourself.org

First Aid Yourself
Essential Breast Cancer Websites

by Betsy Dance

with Breast Self Examination from BreastDoc.com by *Deborah Axelrod*, MD, FACS

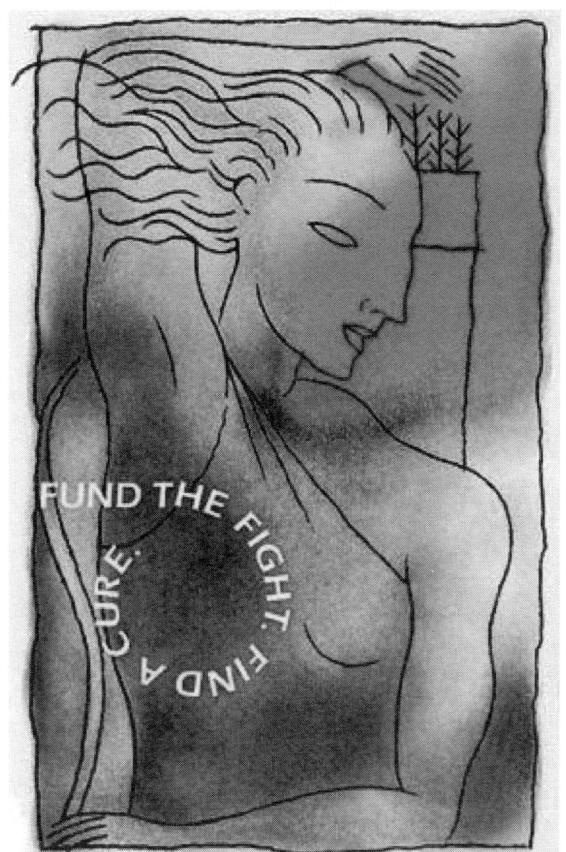

VISIT US ONLINE @ FIRSTAIDYOURSELF.ORG

An original WebPointers™ Interactive Internet Guide
Published by Hope Springs Press

http://www.Webpointers.com

No part of this book may be reproduced or transmitted in any form by any means, electronic or mechanical, including photocopying and recording, or by information storage or retrieval system, except as may be expressly permitted in the 1976 United States Copyright Act or in writing from the publisher.
Requests for permission should be addressed in writing to
Hope Springs Press, 500 Hope Springs Lane, Manakin-Sabot, VA 23103,
or by email to:
Publisher@firstaidyourself.org

Cover Illustration from the semipostal Breast Cancer Research stamp ©1998
U.S. Postal Service. Reproduced with permission. All rights reserved.

Examining Your Own Breasts © 2000, Deborah Axelrod, M.D. Reproduced from
http://www.breastdoc.com with permission. All rights reserved.

Printed in the United States of America
© 2000 Hope Springs Press Inc
All rights reserved.

ISBN 0-9639531-8-4

Library of Congress Catalogue Card Number - 00-105031

OAKWOOD ARTS AND SCIENCES CHARITABLE TRUST SPECIAL EDITION

Editor's Note

This book is not intended to substitute for the care and attention of a trained physician. It is, however, intended to empower those who want to help in the treatment of this disease. If you, or someone you know, suspects breast cancer please begin with a proper medical examination. Early detection is the first step in treatment. The sooner treatment begins, the better your chances for a successful outcome.

You will want to be informed. Your physician will want you to be informed. A series of decisions will have to be made in rapid succession. The more information that can be gathered that is specific to your symptoms and presentation the better will be the quality of the decisions reached. This is where you can help.

The creation of the Internet and the World Wide Web has brought us the blessing of virtually unlimited information. The dark side of this blessing is that the information is rapidly expanding, poorly organized and sometimes difficult to evaluate even if you are a trained medical professional; unlimited information often means unlimited confusion. This book does not purport to have all the answers or to have eliminated confusion. It does, however, offer a model for navigating through the Web to find the information that you can use. Throughout this book Websites are identified by *italics* within the text and listed on the bottom of each right-hand page with the Web address. In the eBook all those Web addresses are active hyperlinks. Move your computer's mouse over the link; when the cursor changes to a webpointer you can click on it and go directly to the Website.

First and foremost, however, this is a story. It is the story of how one friend, who did not have breast cancer, helped another, who did.

It is the story of how she went out onto the World Wide Web and sought information, exploring both popular and virtually unknown Websites, seeking anything and everything that might be of possible benefit. The information she gathered was shared by patient, physician, family and friends in a team effort to guide her treatment and restore her health.

You can do the same. First aid yourself.

In honor of breast cancer patients and their families
with gratitude and appreciation
for their courage, inspiration and leadership.

This Special Edition is made possible by
the generous support of

OAKWOOD ARTS AND SCIENCES CHARITABLE TRUST

FIRST AID YOURSELF— ESSENTIAL BREAST CANCER WEBSITES

Contents

Don't Miss the Hyperlinks 4
Illustrating Courage, Strength & Will 12
Premium Pricing—A Bodacious Idea 14

Introduction 18

Diagnosis: Breast Cancer 20
Sharing Survivors' Stories and Wisdom 22
Connecting to the Web 24
Choosing your Doctor and Hospital 26
Learning the Odds of Beating the Odds 28
Researching Clinical Trials 30
Scouring the Medical Literature 32
Keeping Help Flowing is Key to Progress 34
Testing for Chemosensitivity 36
Surviving is a Matter of Nutrition 38
Giving Up Your Hair 40
Becoming Acquainted with Survivors 42
Finding Alternative Treatments Online 44
Checking Out The Non-Conventional 46
Keeping on Top of the News 48
Staying Informed for Free 50

Coping with Costs	52
Sharing and Giving Back	54
Finding Other Retreats	56
Remembering to Take Care of Yourself	58
Paying Attention to Drugs	60
Paying Attention to Paying	62
Finding Help Around the Home	64
Saying Good-byes	66
Getting a New Breast—or Not	68
Flying with the Angels	70
Losing and Regaining a Breast	72
Learning to Look for Lymphedema	74
Considering Bone Marrow Transplants	76
Financing a Bone Marrow Transplant	78
Accepting the Prospect of Death	80
Preparing for Menopause	82
Uncovering Male Breast Cancer	84
Investigating Environmental Estrogens	86
Pondering Environmental Carcinogens	88
Taking Action for a Change	90
Hoodwinked!	92

FIRST AID YOURSELF— ESSENTIAL BREAST CANCER WEBSITES

Glossary 95
Website Appendix 102

Additional Resources 108
Examining Your Own Breasts 111
Acronyms 116
Index 117
Acknowledgments 123

Afterwords 128

VISIT US ONLINE @ FIRSTAIDYOURSELF.ORG

Illustrating Courage, Strength & Will

The illustration on the cover is taken from the ground-breaking "semipostal" Breast Cancer Research stamp issued by the United States Postal Service on July 29, 1998.

The stamp, which is sold for 40¢, is valid for the first class postage letter rate, currently 33¢. The 7¢ premium is devoted to breast cancer research: 70% to the National Institutes of Health, 30% to the Medical Research Program of the Department of Defense. The first U.S. stamp in history to have net proceeds above the cost of postage earmarked for research organizations, the "semipostal" was the brainchild of Dr. Balazs "Ernie" Bodai, Chief of Surgery for Kaiser Foundation Hospitals in Sacramento, California.

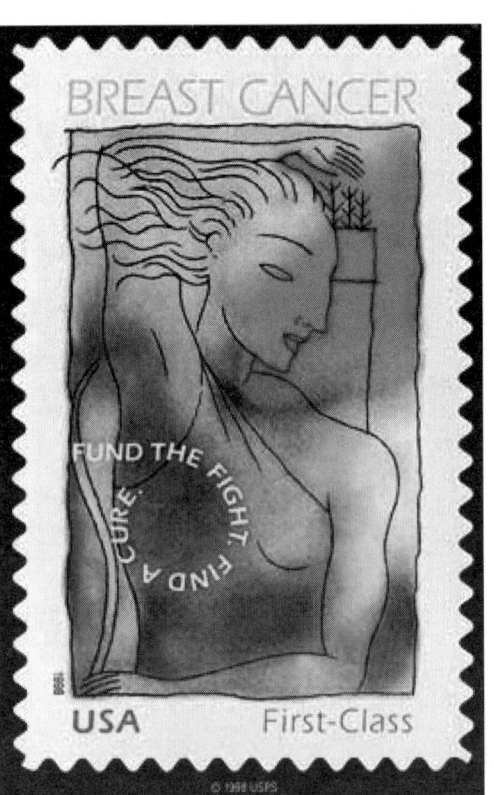

Stamp Design ©1998 U.S. Postal Service. Reproduced with permission. All rights reserved.

By the end of July, 2000, more than 195 million stamps had been sold, generating more than $14 million for research. Special congressional legislation, again spearheaded by Dr. Bodai, was introduced by Senators Diane Feinstein of California and Kay Bailey Hutchison of Texas and quickly gained 63 co-sponsors in the US Senate and 117 co-sponsors in the House of Representatives. An extraordinary lobbying effort, led by Betsy Mullen of WIN Against Breast Cancer, resulted in an unprecedented two-year extension of the semi-postal.

In creating the illustration for the Breast Cancer Research stamp, Baltimore illustrator Whitney Sherman chose classic mythology's goddess of the hunt—Artemis to the Greeks, Diana to the Romans—to represent the ingenuity, strength and will with which women throughout the ages have survived the perils of the natural world.

"Much like the classic Artemis, my modern interpretation wears a quiver and uses arrows to target the disease," Sherman explained. "She is positioned, ready to draw the arrow, her arm raised over her head in a position reminiscent of the one every woman assumes in order to prepare for a self-examination or mammogram. The body is a kaleidoscope of color that defies the boundary of figure, and bursts

FIRST AID YOURSELF— ESSENTIAL BREAST CANCER WEBSITES

outward in an expression of the spirit of each woman's claim to health, hope and strength. The image is a call to action for every woman."

Describing the artistic challenge, Sherman said she developed images that demonstrated courage, strength, hope and spirit. Still she felt a lack.

"One element was missing," said Sherman. "It was the heroic nature of the care-givers, the doctors and the researchers involved in the fight against breast cancer, most importantly it was the women. They are the reason the care-givers give, the doctors doctor and the researchers research. By representing the spirit of those who have fought and are fighting breast cancer, I could speak about the disease."

It is this keen insight that made us feel compelled to reproduce her illustration; we gratefully acknowledge the USPS for its permission to do so.

We encourage you to purchase the Breast Cancer Research semipostal stamps for your own personal or organization's use. Ask for them at your local post office or order them online from the USPS's StampsOnline Website.

StampsOnline   (http://www.stampsonline.com/feature/breast_cancer/cancer.htm)

"One element was missing," said Sherman. "It was the heroic nature of the care-givers, the doctors and the researchers involved in the fight against breast cancer, most importantly it was the women.

Premium Pricing—A Bodacious Idea

The inspired example of Dr. Ernie Bodai and his two-year campaign, involving 15 transcontinental flights, to lobby the U.S. Congress for the creation of the 40¢ semipostal Breast Cancer Research Stamp gave us the idea for this eBook's Premium Pricing program.

This book retails for $14.95.

It also sells for $15.95.

The idea of asking people to pay more than the regular price for an eBook—especially in this Internet age of steep discounting—seemed crazy when we first considered it, but the more we thought about it, the more it began to make sense.

If you volunteer to pay the $15.95 premium price, your extra $1 will be contributed to breast cancer prevention research. But your $1 will also be matched by a $1 contribution from the publisher and another $1 from the distributor, creating a $3 contribution, tripling the impact of your generosity.

The first recipient of Premium Pricing contributions is the Cancer Research Foundation of America (CRFA), a national nonprofit health organization whose mission is the prevention of cancer through scientific research and education. Founded in 1985 by Carolyn Aldigé, the organization's commitment is fueled by the fact that certain cancers are preventable through lifestyle changes, yet more than 550,000 Americans die from the disease annually.

One of only 10 non-federal agencies whose grant review process is approved by the National Institutes of Health, CRFA strengthens the area of cancer prevention research through their grant and fellowship program. Since 1985, CRFA has funded more than 200 scientists at more than 100 leading universities and medical centers.

Over the past 15 years CRFA has awarded more than $36 million in grants to both promising young investigators and established investigators. These investments have helped fund more than 200 basic and applied biomedical research and education projects. CRFA has agreed to direct all contributions raised from sales of the book to breast cancer prevention research.

But there's more. Since we announced our Premium Pricing program and asked other online Websites to become Charter Affiliates in selling the eBook edition, a number have volunteered to donate their full sales commissions as well. They've formed a league of "Hundred Percenters"

We think it's a bold and audacious idea, one that can help bring us another step closer to "Funding the fight—finding a cure."

who contribute all their earnings from the sale of *First Aid Yourself* to CRFA. You'll find them listed at the First Aid Yourself Website and we encourage you to let your friends know about their generosity.

We think Premium Pricing is a bold and audacious idea, one that can help bring us another step closer to "Funding the fight—finding a cure." Early 19th Century Americans combined "bold" and "audacious" to coin a new word for such ideas. They called it "bodacious." We can only imagine they must have had in mind someone like Ernie Bodai.

Thanks, Ernie.

Dr. Ernie Bodai (http://www.kaiserpermanente.org/medicine/permjournal/sum98pjcover.html)
Cancer Research Foundation of America (http://www.crfa.org)
First Aid Yourself (http://www.firstaidyourself.org)

VISIT US ONLINE @ FIRSTAIDYOURSELF.ORG

With love to my goddaughter,
Stafford Olivia Sommers Grayson,
and to her mother, my friend,
Ellen Lea Hickey Grayson.

Introduction

Ellen Lea Hickey Grayson wanted a baby, although that may not be the best place to start.

Perhaps the beginning ought to be our beginnings, as children growing up in a close community in Michigan. We were both born in 1960. Our parents socialized with what seemed to all involved children like fierce abandon. Our parents' fraternity threw Ellen and me together, but it didn't stick until almost 30 years later when we found ourselves near each other; I was living in Washington, D.C., she across the Potomac in Alexandria, Virginia.

My mother died in 1993. She had suffered from lung cancer for a little over a year.

For me, it was an awful, ground-breaking, mystical experience. After she died, I didn't want to leave Michigan where my father remained and my brothers were also lingering. Going back to Washington meant heading into a lonely environment where no one could possibly fathom what had just happened.

Ellen had lost a parent to cancer, too. Her father. By the time we got together we had both come closer to being our own selves. She supported me as I came to terms with my mother's death and my return to Washington.

Perhaps these threads are the natural beginning of this story about how her dance with cancer drew us closer together, but the baby she so longed for seems more right.

Getting pregnant may have put her life in jeopardy. Being a mother made that risk worthwhile. I will start this story with the baby.

Ellen and her husband, Roger, wanted to have a baby in 1994 or so. It turned out to be harder than they had hoped. They chose in vitro fertilization, which, ultimately, was successful.

First, though, there were the shots. Fertility drugs. Mega-doses of hormones. The harvesting of eggs. As she and Roger embarked on this path, they faced agonizing ethical questions such as: if four eggs are harvested and successfully fertilized, do we have quadruplets or abort three viable candidates?

It was an emotional roller-coaster. Of course. Everyone expected that. They were as prepared for it as anyone could be. What no one expected or even thought about—not Ellen, not her husband, not her OB-GYN, not any doctor she'd seen previously and revisited—was that

Getting pregnant may have put her life in jeopardy. Being a mother made that risk worthwhile. I will start this story with the baby.

medical literature was pointing out that young women who had received radiation therapy for Hodgkin's disease were developing breast cancer.

Ellen had had Hodgkin's, a cancer, in 1986. It was stage II—totally survivable. She received three months of radiation. Between the conclusion of her treatment for Hodgkin's and the initiation of her efforts to get pregnant, doctors had learned that secondary breast cancers were popping up in young women who had been radiated for Hodgkin's. To complicate matters further, no one linked this fact with the growing suspicion that fertility drugs pushed up women's estrogen levels—another risk factor for breast cancer.

Problems with Ellen's right breast started almost immediately after Stafford Olivia Sommers Grayson, the miracle baby, was born in June, 1998. Nursing Stafford was painful. Ellen's breasts were loaded with milk that seemed to be backing up and hardening, especially in her right breast. Doctors, midwives, lactation specialists all said the same thing: mastitis. Pump more. Pump less. Cracked, bleeding nipple and dense mass in her right breast notwithstanding—it will pass.

Nearly six months passed before anyone raised a red flag. In December of 1998, she showed her breast to her younger sister. Her sister recommended an acupuncturist, who said, "That is an unusual presentation. You need to see a medical doctor."

Things started moving fast. The breast surgeon took one look and said "Why don't we biopsy this right now?"

When the results of the biopsy came back, the doctors were saying a lot more than unusual presentation. They were saying inflammatory breast cancer (ibc).

The months that followed are not at all blurred. They are a well-documented trail of fear, urgency, research, sacrifice, doctors' appointments, drugs, pain, courage, enlightenment and reward—some of the benefit of which is in this book.

At the beginning of the new year, new century, new millennium, Ellen's breast was gone ... so also the cancer. Stafford was walking and talking. Roger declared the horizontal scar that replaced Ellen's breast "pretty cool." Ellen's mother, primary caregiver, was relieved and exhausted. Her sisters and brother were pleased and predictably anxious. Most importantly, Ellen was alive.

This book is not for someone like Ellen. It is for someone like myself, someone who wants to help—unabashedly help—someone like Ellen stay alive and well.

Things started moving fast. The breast surgeon took one look and said "Why don't we biopsy this right now?"

VISIT US ONLINE @ FIRSTAIDYOURSELF.ORG

Diagnosis: Breast Cancer

8:25 a.m., Saturday, January 17, 1999, Ellen called and dropped a bomb, "I have breast cancer. I found out yesterday. It's inflammatory ductal carcinoma. Can you look on the Internet and find out what that means?" I shook off my paralyzing shock and switched on my computer.

[First, a word of advice: there are frank discussions about lethality and statistics at these Websites. If at all possible, someone other than the person who has just received the cancer diagnosis should do this research.]

It seemed reasonable to start with the standard-bearers—the *National Institutes of Health* (NIH), the *National Cancer Institute* (NCI) and the *American Cancer Society* (ACS).

I started at the National Cancer Institute's Website and stumbled through some press releases and watered-down blather before finding Webpages that really helped.

The most useful address at NCI transported me to a page where, after typing in "inflammatory breast cancer," and hitting the search button, I finally read descriptive news about the cancer challenging Ellen.

At NCI, I also found the *Comprehensive Cancer Database*. "Treatment Summaries for Health Care Professionals" and "Supportive Care Summaries for Health Care Professionals" answered dozens of questions. The former was especially helpful. When I clicked on "Breast Cancer," I got definitions for technical terms and found out how each stage of breast cancer was commonly treated. Supportive Care Summaries discussed symptoms Ellen might face, such as nausea, sleeping problems and mouth sores. Just click on any subject heading for deeper information.

You can do a literature search at NCI, too. I typed in "inflammatory breast cancer," and suddenly had hundreds of articles at my fingertips. Some good. Some bad. All studded with science-jargon, but the more I read, the more familiar I became with medical language. Everything else NCI had could wait.

The NIH Webpage returns a short, timely explanation when you type the name of the cancer you want to learn about into their search engine.

Another behemoth I searched was the University of Pennsylvania's OncoLink site. I found dozens of abstracts, or synopses, of articles that had appeared in credible medical journals.

Then I surfed over to the *American Cancer Society's* (ACS) assessment of complementary and

... the more I read, the more familiar I became with medical language.

alternative treatments. ACS blasts all the "alternative" treatments (those treatments people sometimes pursue *instead* of conventional surgery, chemotherapy and radiation), but mentions some complementary treatments (those used *along with* conventional treatment) with exceedingly faint praise. To see one of the giants, if not endorsing, then at least admitting that Iceland moss could help a cough, or that dried blackberry might have some-mildly-positive-if-not-stronger impact on diarrhea (a common side effect of chemotherapy) encouraged me. At this point I did not know what Ellen thought about complementary treatments. If she were not interested, I thought perhaps her doctors' support might convince her to investigate parallel strategies such as nutrition. Little did I know how fully she would embrace complementary approaches.

After a mind-numbing journey through the heavy hitters' statistics, Dr. David Hankins' site, *International Cancer Alliance for Research and Education* (ICARE), boosted my spirits enormously. His emphasis on living felt like coming home to a puppy. He is a molecular biologist who has taught at Vanderbilt University Medical School, worked for the National Cancer Institute, and directed research projects at Johns Hopkins Medical School.

In fact, ICARE is a good place to start, if you are facing a cancer diagnosis alone, and need a gentle hand to guide you through this jungle.

I ordered Hankins' free report, Cancer Therapy Review, about the cancer that interested me and sent a donation in return.

As Hankins once said: "We want you to have confidence that you are not going to die..."

Go there. It is good medicine.

National Cancer Institute (http://www.nci.nih.gov)
NCI description of disease (http://rex.nci.nih.gov/PATIENTS/SITES_TYPES.html)
NCI disease summaries (http://cancernet.nci.nih.gov/pdq.htm)
NCI literature search (http://cnetdb.nci.nih.gov/cancerlit.shtml)
National Institutes of Health (http://www.nih.gov)
University of Pennsylvania's OncoLink cancer site (http://oncolink.upenn.edu)
American Cancer Society (http://www.cancer.org)
ACS's assessment of complementary and alternative treatments
    (http://www.cancer.org/alt_therapy/index.html)
International Cancer Alliance for Research and Education (http://www.icare.org)

"We want you to have confidence that you are not going to die..."

Sharing Survivors' Stories and Wisdom

After searching through the traditional sites, I found a treasure trove of information I was thrilled to relay to Ellen. The Web is loaded with sites developed by people who have survived cancer and, upon recovery share what they have learned with others facing a similar struggle. This meant two things: first, there was some good information out there from people with experience, and second, there were survivors galore.

Dozens of exceptional people have developed extraordinary Websites designed to help others navigate their way, online, through a cancer diagnosis and the difficulties of the disease. Who better to learn from than from someone who has received the same diagnosis—and even better, survived it? These generous survivors were going to help us get through our ignorance of medical terminology and also through the unsettling sense of urgency that often follows a cancer diagnosis.

The very best sites provide free, concise information and answer questions only those who have been through cancer would think to ask. The creators of these sites have a common mission to make things easier for others in similar situations. I was lucky enough to find some good sites quickly.

Cancer survivor Alexandra Andrews developed *Cancerlinks*, a site with multiple addresses leading to the same of the Web location. If you can't reach one of them, try one of the others. The information is available in eight different languages. Find the cancer you need to learn about, then double-click on that box to go to more specialized information. You will be taken to a new page with specific links to a broad range of Websites—general medical information; advocacy and legislation; caregivers; online support groups—each of which offers fairly targeted information.

Cancerlinks also has a useful Web tutorial.

Be forewarned, no matter where or how you start, the vastness of the Web can appear to be overwhelming. Working consistently and persistently however, you will get a handle on what you're trying to understand.

If you need a good description of "staging" or "grading," check *Steve Dunn's Cancer Guide*. He's a cancer survivor.

This meant two things: first, there was some good information out there from people with experience, and second, there were survivors galore.

FIRST AID YOURSELF— ESSENTIAL BREAST CANCER WEBSITES

After you have answered some of your own questions about the diagnosis, Virginia Hetrick's site, *You Are Not Alone* (YANA) is excellent. Hetrick is very much alive eight years after her diagnosis of inflammatory breast cancer. Strictly speaking, YANA is a high-dose chemotherapy support group, but much of the information is useful and relevant for anyone dealing with cancer. The site addresses many of the nuts and bolts concerns, fears, and too-often-unspoken requirements of any cancer patient.

I clicked my way through the whole site and found sensible diet recommendations based on research from over 4,500 studies, as well as serious science-based articles, descriptions, and definitions: "Seminal articles on high-dose chemotherapy"; "Getting your gut back" after chemo; "What happens when the insurance won't pay?"; "Stressbusters: things we do to help cope"; "Dealing with work issues"; and two of the most helpful, "What ARE those blood tests?" and "Organizing your medical records." Many of these articles are tucked away in "Patients' Perspectives," and the subjects change so you may not see these specific articles, but you will probably find articles of interest.

There is also a very funny log of Hetrick's personal, day-to-day, year-by-year experience with cancer. Her lightheartedness in the face of such a devastating situation humbled me into remembering that one of the best ways to get through the darkness of the hard days is to invoke its most spirited rival—humor.

Unlike so many sites on the Internet, YANA is mercifully self-contained. The information is unsentimental and on-point. Should you need them, and you will, YANA offers links to other important Websites.

One more thing that will help in the early days is NCI's site that gives a list of their *designated cancer centers*. Now try and get a good night's sleep. Tomorrow the battle will rage on.

Cancerlist (http://www.acor.org/Cancerlist)
Cancerlinks.org (http://www.cancerlinks.org)
Steve Dunn's Cancer Guide (http://www.cancerguide.org)
You Are Not Alone (YANA) (http://www.yana.org)
National Cancer Institute's designated Cancer Centers
    (http://www.nci.nih.gov/cancercenters/centers1.htmv)

... one of the best ways to get through the darkness of the hard days is to invoke its most spirited rival—humor.

VISIT US ONLINE @ FIRSTAIDYOURSELF.ORG

Connecting to the Web

Washington is a busy town. The telephone is a major player and Ellen and I had made great use of it during the six or so years after we had reconnected following my mother's death. We shared many interests. Ellen writes. She paints. She reads. She taught college. She had invited me over to dinner and I met her husband, Roger. Our friendship blossomed and continued to grow.

When email came along I begged her to connect to the Internet, to log on, to get up to speed, but she and Roger opted not to.

Weeks before her breast cancer diagnosis, Ellen and Roger had moved into a fine new house big enough to accommodate Stafford's life. Overnight moving boxes vanished; walls were painted; books and photographs appeared; fabrics were chosen; furniture was placed and draperies were hung. The house was transformed. It looked like they had lived in it forever. Nobody who witnessed this non-spectacle could believe it. Suddenly they were hosting a party in honor of Stafford's christening when they barely had their new phone system hooked up. Then Ellen was told she was sick.

She and Roger relented and got the extra phone line for the computer. Ellen started using email and found it kept her connected when she didn't feel like taking phone calls. Her brother had a Webpage developed for her. She started posting photographs and journal entries that have kept friends and family informed about each step of her path and progress.

The Web became a lifeline for Ellen, but not everyone has Internet access or a computer with Internet capability. Not everyone can simply haul in a new phone line when they want it. At the turn of the century half of America's households still didn't have Web access. However, lots of public facilities offer public access. One call to your local public library will tell you if you can surf the 'net there. The same goes for universities. More and more hospitals offer their patients access. If all those avenues fail, try a cybercafe—one of those trendy urban coffee bars that have computers and Internet access at every booth.

There are thousands of cybercafés to choose from, as Ernst Larsen points out in his book, "*Internet Cafe Guide*," available on the Web and written for travelers who cannot stand to be away from their email one minute longer. It lists, by Internet and street address, 2,000 Internet cafes in 113 countries, from Sri Lanka to South Africa to Nepal and all across the U.S.

Ellen started using email and found it kept her connected when she didn't feel like taking phone calls.

In case Larsen didn't get every last cybercafe in his book, Dutch native and U.S.A.-traveler Harrie Meeuwissen developed his own *cybercafe list* presented alphabetically by state. Meeuwissen is just an ordinary person, just a traveler, but his site covers a lot of territory and it's easy to use.

If a cybercafe doesn't work, there are other options. You can find access at many Kinko's, Mail Boxes Etc., Touchnet Kiosks, iCom Networks, Atcom-Iport Cyberbooths, GTE Cyberbooths, Sky Links, Business Anywhere, Club Disney and also at many hotels. I pulled all that from The Cybercafe Search Engine that mentions other public access points located around the world. The page is part of a vast ring of cybercafe sites and is updated frequently.

The rapid development and marketing of ever-more-powerful, personal computers has led to a growing supply of slightly less-powerful but still fully-functional, second-hand computers at relatively low prices. A handful of companies such as Spinway.com have now pioneered *free Internet access* without monthly fees.

More recently, a new breed of machines that are solely designed for email and Web use (known as *Internet Appliances*) such as the "i-Opener" have been introduced for as little as $99.

The point is, your circumstances don't have to limit your access to the Web and the information you need. If you aren't yet able to establish your own Internet connection there are alternatives.

Ernst Larsen's "Internet Cafe Guide" (http://www.netcafeguide.com)
Harrie Meeuwissen's cybercafe list (http://usa.dedas.com/cybcaf.html)
Free Internet Access (http://www.spinway.com)
Internet Appliance iOpener (http://www.netpliance.com)

For a fuller list of Public Internet access locations (http://cybercaptive.com/pia.shtml)

If you aren't yet able to establish your own Internet connection there are alternatives.

VISIT US ONLINE @ FIRSTAIDYOURSELF.ORG

Choosing your Doctor and Hospital

After her diagnosis, Ellen went to the doctor who had treated her Hodgkin's, the one who neglected to mention her high risk for breast cancer. Upon seeing her swollen and painful breast and learning of her breast cancer diagnosis, he said, discouragingly, "The world is a cesspool." He sent her to an oncologist at Georgetown University Hospital, but the hospital's narrow focus on research made Ellen uncomfortable. She wanted an oncologist who clearly believed in her life and who was open to complementary treatments.

The *University of Texas MD Anderson Cancer Center* specializes in inflammatory breast cancer. I hoped she would move. Ellen didn't want cancer to take over her life or disrupt Stafford's.

Following different leads, she traipsed from one oncologist to the next, waiting to fall in love with someone who would help her keep her life. Finally, she found Dr. Carolyn Hendricks, an oncologist in nearby Chevy Chase, Maryland, with the perfect combination of outlook and experience.

Ultimately, Ellen chose an aggressive protocol developed by Dr. Clifford Hudis at Memorial Sloan-Kettering Cancer Center in New York. Dr. Hendricks would administer the chemotherapeutic drugs in Washington so Ellen wouldn't have to move.

During this frantic time, I read Laura Landro's book, "Survivor, Taking Control of Your Fight Against Cancer" about her own experience with leukemia. Landro, a Wall Street Journal reporter, emphasizes asking questions and choosing your own treatment instead of being bullied or intimidated by your doctors. A handful of phone numbers and Internet addresses in the book helped me find *Best Doctors*—an organization that, for a fee, helps patients find medical care tailored to their specific needs, using a worldwide database of physicians. I wanted Ellen to sign up immediately. Instead, she designed a medical team herself that let her stay home while benefitting from some of the best medical advice and attention available in the world.

But Best Doctors is still a viable, though expensive, option. You can read about it on the Internet, but if you want to participate, you can call: 888-DOCTORS.

There are other sites to research, as well. The Complete Internet Medical Resource Doctor's Guide has an alphabetical list of Web addresses for hospitals around the world.

The *P/S/L NuMedia* group, sponsored by pharmaceutical companies from around the world, also provides a list of hospital Webpages.

Landro emphasizes asking questions and choosing your own treatment instead of being bullied or intimidated by your doctors.

26

An Original WebPointers™ Interactive Internet Guide © 2000 Hope Springs Press Inc

FIRST AID YOURSELF— ESSENTIAL BREAST CANCER WEBSITES

Drug Infonet, is similar, but lists different hospitals. Their alphabetical list includes each hospital's location on the same page. Hospital Webpage quality varies widely. Some are simple address and phone listings, others are more helpful. Most just barely mask the fact that health care has become big business.

CenterWatch was developed to help patients find relevant, industry-sponsored clinical trials; their Website has a state-by-state list of hospitals specializing in oncology.

Martindale's Health Science Guide is another treasure trove of data. Here, you can launch a search for hospitals worldwide, hospitals in the U.S., or hospitals by country. It is maintained by John Lester, in the Department of Neurology, at Massachusetts General Hospital, and has no connection to the well-known legal directory.

To look for doctors, you can either begin at Martindale's site, or go straight to the American Medical Association's (AMA) *Online Doctor Finder*. Once there, you must first agree not to hold the AMA liable for decisions based on the information at the site. Don't let that scare you off— accept their terms and enter. You may then either type in a doctor's name or a medical specialty, such as "oncology." Searching a doctor's name will turn up where he or she went to school and did a residency as well as a current location and phone number.

Finding the right doctors and the right hospital went a long way toward putting Ellen's mind at ease. That it had to happen first, when she was least educated about her situation, complicated the process enormously. But she did it. You can too.

University of Texas MD Anderson Cancer Center (http://www.mdanderson.org)
Best Doctors (http://www.bestdoctors.com)
The P/S/L NuMedia Group's Complete Internet Medical Resource Doctor's Guide
    (http://www.pslgroup.com/dg/hospsite.htm)
Drug Infonet (http://www.druginfonet.com/hospital.htm)
CenterWatch (http://www.centerwatch.com/PROCAT12.HTM)
Martindale's Health Science Guide's doctors/hospital search
    (http://sun2.lib.uci.edu/HSG/Pharmacy.html#DOCHOS)
John Lester's hospital search page (http://neurowww2.mgh.harvard.edu/hospitalWebusa.html)
AMA's doctor search page (http://www.ama-assn.org/iwcf/iwcfmgr206/aps?2331732074)

... you must first agree not to hold the AMA liable for decisions based on the information at the site. Don't let that scare you off—accept their terms and enter.

An Original WebPointers™ Interactive Internet Guide © 2000 Hope Springs Press Inc

27

Learning the Odds of Beating the Odds

There was a message from Ellen on my phone machine. Her voice was low and shaky. She'd been to see another doctor who had told her statistics about ibc. They are very grim.

Ellen spoke slowly. "Every new thing I hear is worse than what I heard before. The news is overwhelming me," she said. "I am scared."

For a long time after that, Ellen didn't want to hear about "the odds," but it's hard information to shut out when you spend your days with oncologists. Doctor after doctor pointed to statistic after statistic from study after study that had nothing whatsoever to do with Ellen. It *was* scary. Eighty per cent of people who get ibc, said the doctors, don't live past five years. How do you trust your doctor enough to take advice, yet disregard predictions about life span?

I believe that statistics are for doctors, not for survivors. Although I tried hard to convince her to see that, it was a tough sell. Ellen wasn't about to accept my view of things. She had to believe it herself before it could come true.

Even if they're good, hearing or reading about statistics is depressing, and I guarantee you that someone, somewhere along the line, is going to start hammering them home. Oncology must be a tough field.

The date of death is something else some oncologists sometimes forecast. As if they know. Some patients demand a forecast, no matter how inexact or discouraging. Others don't want to hear an educated guess. Of course, if you don't want a forecast, the knowledge that one may be available must loom on your horizon like a dreadful gathering storm. Doctors need a lot of training in this area.

Keeping the emphasis on life seems more reasonable if living is what you want to do. That can be difficult when the doctors go on and on about how bleak the whole situation is and how poor the chances are that you'll live much past breakfast.

But every day someone is beating the odds. *Cancer-Free Connections* is all about living. It's about beating the odds. Stories. Strategies. Resources. Names—some famous and surprising—of people who lived straight through the diagnosis and treatment and experienced a complete remission or are now free of the disease. It's for and about people who live with cancer. While this disease is not always a death sentence, it does always promise to be an immense inconvenience.

> *"Every new thing I hear is worse than what I heard before. The news is overwhelming me," she said. "I am scared."*

FIRST AID YOURSELF— ESSENTIAL BREAST CANCER WEBSITES

One of the statistics I pulled from this site says, "Half of those diagnosed with cancer this year will live out their normal life span." That buoyant piece of news came from the City of Hope National Medical Center. It brought to mind Alice Roosevelt Longworth, terror of Washington society, who after a double-mastectomy, described herself as "the only topless hostess in D.C." She died on February 20, 1980, eight days after her 96th birthday.

Tom Marron, who struggled through melanoma, created Cancer-Free Connections for the obvious reasons. He's loaded it with survivor anecdotes from the likes of Julia Child, Michael Milken, Robert Goulet, Norman Schwarzkopf and others, as well as including details about books, magazines and videos geared toward living.

The Website's *inspiration page* is stocked with quote after quote from person after person who was supposed to be a dead statistic and is instead a living one.

At some point after Ellen started treatment, we went to talk with a prominent oncologist at a prominent oncology center at a prominent university hospital about bone marrow transplants. The woman was significantly overweight and had a nasty skin rash. She gravely yet breezily told Ellen that because she'd had radiation for Hodgkin's, she did not qualify for a bone marrow transplant at this particular hospital even if she wanted one.

The drive home began in relative silence.

"I hate to say this, Bets," Ellen finally said, "but how seriously can I take a doctor who appears to be in much worse health than I am, especially when she's basing my chances of survival on what, at some point, happened inside some petri dish?"

With that, I knew Ellen had become a believer in her own life.

Cancer-Free Connections (http://www.cancer-free.com)
Inspiration page (http://www.cancer-free.com/secrets.htm#psychology)

The site's inspiration page is stocked with quote after quote from person after person who was supposed to be a dead statistic and is instead a living one.

An Original WebPointers™ Interactive Internet Guide © 2000 Hope Springs Press Inc

Researching Clinical Trials

Shortly after Ellen was diagnosed, she realized the most important part of the diagnosis was the *inflammatory* part. Shortly after that, she learned there might be "liver involvement" —the potential for the metastatic spread of cancer cells to other organs. That would mean stage IV cancer: the worst.

Of these developments, she said, "The inflammatory part was bad; I figured I could handle that. But a liver metastasis? I'm going to need God to get through that."

God is said to move in mysterious ways. For some, God's involvement may take the form of a clinical trial—the leading edge of research where new drugs and treatments are tested before being approved for general use. If you are interested, and can get help from your oncologist in finding an appropriate clinical trial, take it. If that help is not forthcoming, begin your own research while keeping your oncologist informed.

Clinical trials are going on all over the country and are funded by a variety of sponsors: hospitals, drug companies, the National Cancer Institute—the list goes on. It is not uncommon for a patient's legwork to turn up the most successful route to remission and survival.

Before digging in, I read cancer survivor Steve Dunn's evenhanded and valuable *write-up of clinical trials*. He swears by them; one saved his life.

The *National Library of Medicine* recently created a registry under a mandate from Congress. When I looked approximately 4,000 studies, pulled from 47,000 sites, were listed. Typing "inflammatory breast cancer" into a search field, I got information on 14 ibc-related clinical trials. Clicking on just one I found an explanation of the purpose of the trial, objectives, treatment outline, eligibility criteria, location and principal contact; to my surprise, it was Dr. Clifford A. Hudis, Ellen's primary oncologist at Memorial Sloan-Kettering Hospital.

It helps to know that the *National Cancer Institute* (NCI) funds a handful of cooperative research organizations that perform trials across the country. Each Website has a different format and offers varying degrees of information, so don't expect this to be a breeze. Also, most of the NCI cooperatives have password-protected areas available only for members. I felt the best information was being kept from me, but if you hunt diligently and make phone calls when you have questions—and talk with your oncologist—you will probably find what you need.

To see what the various cooperatives have to offer, check each individual address. When you

It is not uncommon for a patient's legwork to turn up the most successful route to remission and survival.

look at the *National Surgical Adjuvant Breast and Bowel Project,* below the heading, "The NSABP Protocols Open For Accrual," you will see a few number/letter combinations. Click on each to see more about the clinical trials they represent.

NCI conducts trials elsewhere, too. NCI is vast, but a handful of addresses, listed below, will get you started. When I visited their Bethesda campus Website, I typed "breast cancer" into the search field and got information on 58 trials. Each listed trial had a link to either more substantive information about the trial or a short bio on the doctor in charge.

NCI also oversees a site that tells you about *high priority trials being conducted outside NCI*. They have a clinical trials update page, and a page that shows a map of the U.S.A. where you can click on any state and zoom in to the nearest NCI-funded cancer center.

For clinical trials research, the University of Pennsylvania's *OncoLink* was my last stop. Straightforward and easy to use, it is a relief after slogging through the NCI sites.

I typed in Breast Cancer and turned up a list of 17 studies. Lo and behold, there was a study for women with a prior diagnosis of Hodgkin's Disease who contracted secondary breast cancer from the Hodgkin's radiation—exactly what happened to Ellen.

Searching for clinical trials used to be frustrating work. Now, thanks to the clinical trial registry, physicians, researchers and patients can find each other quickly—and that's important when minutes matter.

>   Steve Dunn's write-up of clinical trials (http://www.cancerguide.org/clinical_trials.html)
>   National Library of Medicine's clinical trial registry (http://clinicaltrials.gov)
>   The National Surgical Adjuvant Breast and Bowel Project
>   (http://www.nsabp.pitt.edu/NSABP_Protocols.html)
>   National Cancer Institute
>   Overview (http://cancertrials.nci.nih.gov/NCI_CANCER_TRIALS/zones/TrialInfo/Finding)
>   Trials at the Bethesda, Maryland Campus (http://www-dcs.nci.nih.gov/clin_trials)
>   High priority trials outside NCI (http://cancertrials.nci.nih.gov)
>   Updates (http://cancertrials.nci.nih.gov/NCI_CANCER_TRIALS/zones/PressInfo/updates.html)
>   To find an NCI-funded cancer center
>   (http://cancertrials.nci.nih.gov/NCI_CANCER_TRIALS/zones/TrialInfo/Finding/centers/html/map.html)
>   University of Pennsylvania's OncoLink (http://www.oncolink.upenn.edu/clinical_trials/protocols.html)

Lo and behold, there was a study for women with a prior diagnosis of Hodgkin's Disease who contracted secondary breast cancer from the Hodgkin's radiation—exactly what happened to Ellen.

Scouring the Medical Literature

"Look," Dr. Hendricks said to Ellen, "if it's stage IV, it's going to be extremely tough. If it's stage III, you have a real chance." Dr. Hendricks closed the book she'd been pointing in. Ellen sat so still I thought she might not be breathing.

"I'm sorry to tell you this," Hendricks said. "You've seen three oncologists already and if this is the first time you are hearing this news, well, shame on them." Prior to breast cancer, Ellen did not—or could not—cry. That has changed. She wept openly as she took in this new information.

Long before Ellen's diagnosis, I had planned to leave Washington in January and move west. Our friend, F.K., whom we had known since childhood, would drive out with me. When I found a place to live, he would visit as often as his job allowed. He and I were in love. Snags in my plan, however, had kept me in Washington, so I was still there when Ellen's cancer was diagnosed. By mid-January, instead of being in the foothills of New Mexico's Sangre de Cristo range, I was sitting amongst mountains of medical articles.

There is a lot to be gained from reading medical literature. You can find out who is active in the field, where they practice, what they write, study, and think. So much new information is being developed every day no one can be expected to stay on top of it all the time. It shouldn't be surprising that some cancer patients have saved themselves by tracking down research their doctors initially overlooked or had been unaware of.

Although I have no medical training, I knew enough to understand the statistics. I had learned about what drugs were commonly used for combating inflammatory breast cancer. Everything I read said ibc was rare and fast. Most sources advised against wasting time on a second opinion and encouraged immediate treatment. I was reading these details before anyone had told Ellen about them.

My role was not to advise Ellen, but to be by her side when she got tough news, and to help her sort through it. Her husband, Roger, would have liked to be there but had to stay at work to finance whatever might be coming down the pike. I agonized over whether or not I should tell her what I'd been reading, but deep down I knew I should not be the one to tell her difficult news. For one thing, she'd have to hear it from a doctor to take it as seriously as she had to and for another, I served best as a buffer. My resolve was shaken frequently.

Medline is a clearinghouse of online information compiled by the National Library of Medi-

Some cancer patients have even saved themselves by tracking research their doctors overlooked.

FIRST AID YOURSELF— ESSENTIAL BREAST CANCER WEBSITES

cine. For direct access to the breast cancer articles, go to PubMed and enter the words "Breast Cancer Treatment." You will get pages and pages of medical abstracts culled from the industry's most respected journals. If you like a particular article, click on the "Related Articles" link next to it. Buying the full text of an article is possible through something called Loansome Doc, which you may join. Click *Loansome Doc* for instructions.

Early on, Ellen devoted her energies to getting herself from one day to the next. She chose not to compromise her strength by taking in more information than she could reasonably handle. Cancer or not, she needed to sleep at night so she could rise at six a.m. to feed her baby. Having someone else around to do some of the reading helped.

For a shortcut to 36 medical journals, go to the American Medical Association *online publications page* with links the Journal of Clinical Oncology, The Lancet, New England Journal of Medicine, Journal of the American Medical Association (JAMA) and Nature—all reputable.

JAMA has a link to current *women's health articles.* There are usually plenty of articles about breast cancer. From there, you can go to Additional Recent Reports and Special Reports (midpage). If you see nothing relevant, use the search option and type in "Breast Cancer." The day I checked, there were 60 articles of general breast cancer interest, dating back to 1996.

Some publications do not offer the full text of some articles unless you subscribe. The New England Journal of Medicine, for example, costs $69 annually. Your doctor may already have it and will probably gladly share.

Another great place to look for reliable articles by respected doctors and researchers is *CancerNet*, a service provided by the National Cancer Institute.

Keep in mind none of the studies you will read factor in the unique circumstances of the person you happen to care about. None of the authors knew Ellen. They had not met Stafford. They did not know Ellen had started painting again after many fallow years. They did not know that, except for the cancer, she was exceptionally healthy.

By the way, when the results came back, she was stage III.

The National Library of Medicine's Medline (http://www.ncbi.nlm.nih.gov/Literature/index.html)
To join Loansome Doc (http://www.ncbi.nlm.nih.gov/PubMed)
AMA's online publications page (http://www.ama-assn.org/med_link/peer.htm)
JAMA's women's health page (http://www.ama-assn.org/special/womh/newsline/newsline.htm)
National Cancer Institute's CancerNet (http://cancernet.nci.nih.gov/clinpdq/canlit/breast.html)

Keep in mind none of the studies you will read factor in the unique circumstances of the person you happen to care about.

VISIT US ONLINE @ FIRSTAIDYOURSELF.ORG

Keeping Help Flowing is Key to Progress

Chemotherapy is a key element of ibc treatment and Ellen's first chemotherapy was on January 28, less than two weeks after her initial diagnosis. Initially, she followed a dose-dense protocol: the highest doses, short of a bone marrow transplant, that could be given without killing her. The doctor administering the drugs had never given such high doses.

What do you say to someone about to start chemotherapy to fight a rare form of breast cancer? I found the answer in an *online group devoted specifically to ibc*. Most participants had ibc, though some were friends, family members or even cancer researchers.

I'd get email from this group and could respond exactly as if I were emailing a friend. After I'd participated for a while, some members actually were like friends.

A few days before Ellen's chemo infusion, I asked the group to send notes to show her she was not alone and that people lived through this. Warm, encouraging responses poured back. On the morning of her chemo, I gave her an armful of love and support tied with a red ribbon.

The ibc list has been invaluable. I have gone to those courageous people many times with delicate questions and have always received informed, generous responses.

Lists such as this serve a critical function these days. Information spreads through them like wildfire. Someone has seen a relevant study or has heard about an especially effective treatment or has fresh advice on how to combat some side effect of the disease or treatment and—presto!—that news is in everyone's hands immediately.

The ibc list was created and is maintained by Pete Bevin and Menya Wolfe. Menya was diagnosed with ibc in 1996. If you are not involved with ibc, other lists exist for other cancers and conditions. Those mentioned here are free.

Joining a list can be depressing. Members are often quite ill and some people die. Also, the volume of mail can be overwhelming. Ellen was a member of the ibc list for a while, but recently signed off. I continue to learn and participate and tell Ellen about anything that seems useful.

The *Association of Cancer Online Resources, Inc.*, (ACOR) is a nonprofit group started in 1996. Funded by donations, it runs cancer-related online discussion groups for patients, caregivers, research scientists and healthcare professionals, and provides good links and information.

Cancer Care, a national nonprofit that has offered emotional and practical support to cancer

The ibc list has been invaluable. I have gone to those courageous people many times with delicate questions and have always received informed, generous responses.

patients and others since 1944, hosts three lists. Their lists are overseen by oncology social workers. To participate, *Cancer Care* asks for three commitments: take part in the online discussion three times a week; stay connected for at least three months; and be willing to fill out a questionnaire at the beginning and end of your participation. If you agree to all this, you will see an email address to contact so you can get access.

CancerHelp connects new cancer patients, their families and friends, to crucial information.

After Ellen received that first infusion, we went to the parking garage to get her car. After a seemingly endless wait, we were told that the car keys, along with a cherished, heart-shaped, silver key-chain Ellen had been given as a bridesmaid several years earlier, had been lost. With that admission, the men who ran the garage stopped speaking English. Ellen and I trucked up and down five flights of stairs and scoured the elevator for her keys. No luck. I feared the fresh chemo in her system was going to make her sick. It did not.

Without keys we could go nowhere. Barely civil, Ellen said to the man in charge, "Look, Sir, I've just had my first shot of chemotherapy for breast cancer, and I need to get home." As our taxis headed off in different directions, I was grateful for all the loving notes, filled with praise and encouragement, she had to read. She had a spare key at home and was able to pick up her car the next day.

When the time came for her next infusion, Ellen picked me up and before she realized where she was, force of habit led her to turn the car into the same negligent parking garage.

"Should we just back out and find another place to park?" she asked.

Before I could answer another car pulled in behind us. We could only go forward.

We got out and the same men we had cursed a week earlier approached us. One beamed at the sight of Ellen and ran into the office, reappearing with Ellen's other keys still latched onto her silver key-chain. A few days after the keys had vanished, another patron turned them in but no one had the Graysons' phone number. They had only hoped she would come back.

Inflammatory Breast Cancer (http://www.bestiary.com/ibc)
Association of Cancer Online Resources, Inc. (http://www.acor.org)
    To subscribe, send an email message to LISTSERV@morgan.ucs.mun.ca.
Cancer Care online support groups (http://www.cancercare.org/services/online3.htm)
CancerHelp online support groups (http://www.rwneill.com/cancerhelp.htm)

I was grateful for all the loving notes, filled with praise and encouragement, she had to read.

VISIT US ONLINE @ FIRSTAIDYOURSELF.ORG

Testing for Chemosensitivity

When Ellen got inflammatory breast cancer, she went public. She wanted people to know. She wanted their prayers, their concern and whatever energy they had to spare. The result was that people prayed for her in churches from Jackson Hole, Wyoming to Grosse Pointe, Michigan to Nashville, Tennessee. Cards and letters clumped up in her mailbox. People called. And people talked about her.

One day a friend called Ellen. She'd heard something about tumor cells being tested with various chemotherapy drugs to see which ones had the highest impact. "Precision Something, someplace in Pennsylvania," the friend said. What, Ellen asked, could I find out about this.

I immediately asked the inflammatory breast cancer online discussion group, and found the procedure was called "chemosensitivity testing." One man's wife had even tried it with good results. Cancer survivor Steve Dunn—the man I mentioned in the clinical trials section—offers a thorough *description of chemosensitivity testing*.

I learned that tumor cells are extracted, sent to a special lab, exposed to chemotherapy drugs and, as Dunn explains, "Drugs that are most effective in killing the cultured cells are recommended for treatment." The caveat—laboratories need fresh tumor cells and the procedure is most effective either before or some time after chemotherapy has been administered.

Precision Therapeutics, in Pittsburgh, uses a patented technique called "ChemoFxAssay" to grow cells from an individual's tumor. Once grown, cells are tested with various drugs.

Founded in 1995 by Dr. Paul. L. Kornblith, Precision Therapeutics is a for-profit biomedical company. He told me it focuses "on the interaction of cultivated tumor cells with chemotherapy and immunology-based drugs." In 1998, the University of Pittsburgh Medical Center teamed up with the company for collaboration.

According to their Webpage: "Precision Therapeutics' capabilities capitalize on opportunities in the rapidly expanding anti-cancer drug market. Growth is supported by increasing cancer rate statistics and significant expansion in the number of FDA approved cancer therapy drugs."

It's a business. The Carnegie Science Center even named Dr. Kornblith the 1998 Entrepreneur of the Year in their Science Category.

If that seems cold, read Dr. Kornblith's professional medical history by clicking "People" on

... people prayed for her in churches from Jackson Hole, Wyoming to Grosse Pointe, Michigan to Nashville, Tennessee.

An Original WebPointers™ Interactive Internet Guide © 2000 Hope Springs Press Inc

FIRST AID YOURSELF— ESSENTIAL BREAST CANCER WEBSITES

the Webpage. He served as Director of Neuro-Oncology at Massachusetts General Hospital, was an assistant professor of surgery at Harvard Medical School, and held a leadership position at the National Institutes of Health. He brings other worthy credentials to the job, too.

By the time we figured out what Precision Therapeutics was, Ellen didn't need it. She'd had her biopsy almost a month earlier and no one was about to risk a new one simply to get fresh cells for chemosensitivity testing. Later on, cells from her mastectomy might be used, but everyone tacitly expected that by then she would not need such measures. In addition, an oncologist had to order the procedure, not the patient or the patient's friend. Ellen hadn't developed a powerful relationship with her oncologist at this point, although we felt sure that if asked, the doctor would order. The good part was that insurance would probably help with the costs.

Rational Therapeutics Cancer Laboratories, based in Long Beach, California, also performs chemosensitivity testing. Patients either go to Long Beach to have the work done, or send a bit of biopsied cell, overnight, to the labs. At Rational Therapeutics, staff will also suggest a "carefully developed antioxidant and nutrition program..." That's a plus. Dr. Robert Nagourney, who heads up Rational Therapeutics, has included his substantial and respectable curriculum vitae on the site, which offers a more in-depth description of chemosensitivity testing than does the newer Precision Therapeutics site.

I ran across Rational Therapeutics on Michael Lerner's Commonweal page, which I will discuss later. Briefly, when Lerner's father had cancer 15 years ago, Lerner toiled to find options. As a result, he established *Commonweal*, a health and environmental research institute.

Since we learned about chemosensitivity testing when it was already too late, the idea went from First Line of Possible Defense to a back pocket, where it remains today. Our unspoken expectation has become reality.

Description of chemosensitivity testing (http://www.cancerguide.org/unconv_conv.html)
Precision Therapeutics in Pittsburgh, Pennsylvania (http://www.ptilabs.com)
Rational Therapeutics Cancer Laboratories (http://www.rational-t.com/index.html)
Commonweal (http://www.commonweal.org)

Since we learned about chemosensitivity testing when it was already too late, the idea went from First Line of Possible Defense to a back pocket, where it remains today.

Surviving is a Matter of Nutrition

Not everyone believes complementary medicine has something to offer cancer patients, but I do. When Ellen was diagnosed, I hoped she would at least look into something besides chemotherapy, surgery and radiation.

As it turned out, she had always been interested in things such as biofeedback and meditation. Cancer inspired her to explore a full range of complementary approaches to good health. She began weekly talks with a spiritual advisor and less frequent visits to a psychic astrologer. She also found a nutritionist, Irv Rosenberg. Irv and his partner, Mickey Weinstein, run the 30-year-old Apothecary Pharmacy in Bethesda, Maryland, and they have worked with others who have cancer.

We met Irv for the first time in his office in Bethesda, Maryland. He talked with us about good fats and bad fats and the benefits of fish oil. He condemned wheat (for Ellen), too much sugar, dairy and most meats. He told Ellen to eat organic foods and to stick with vegetables, soy, legumes and non-wheat grains, and then he recommended she take practically every nutrient capsule on the market and sold them to her through his *Apothecary*.

I didn't like Irv at first, because he seemed so intent on making a buck off Ellen's cancer, but I was wrong. His recommendations improved Ellen's life. True, the quantities of capsules she's taken since January, have challenged her patience and ability to swallow, but the good things she's pumped into her body have kept her body strong and resilient through chemotherapy.

Following Irv's recommendations, Ellen decided she would try not to put another bite of non-organic food into her mouth, nor would she eat one thing that was not on Irv's list of acceptable foods. Consequently, although wonderful foods filled their kitchen (Roger is an excellent cook), Ellen came home from meeting with Irv and had nothing to eat. Irv had just impressed us with the importance of flooding Ellen's system with plenty of good foods. She had to eat and she had to eat that evening. Ellen was shouldering huge psychological burdens already. Now, her kitchen did not have any of the resources she had just been told would help her live. It was a crisis.

Roger and I fanned out through the city to remedy the situation.

By eating organic food, Irv explained, Ellen would avoid pesticides and other toxins. She is lucky to live in an area where choices abound. Organic food is not available in every community,

> *Ellen decided she wouldn't put another bite of non-organic food into her mouth*

but thanks to the Internet, you can order many items and have them delivered to your door.

By visiting just a couple of sites, you can tap into a great variety. *Organic Kitchen* is an "organic foods product, research and marketing company..." that has searched the Internet and provides links to a wide range of organic resources. They list organic restaurants by state. They list sources for organic snacks, soy products, baking goods, rice, prepared foods and more. They list stores—Vegetarian Direct; Rainbow Organics; and To Life Organic Food and Herb Company, an organic, kosher, online market. Your order can be on your doorstep in a matter of days—or even the next day, for a *big* delivery charge.

Yahoo!'s organic food page has a long directory of sources that deliver.

The Green Marketplace sells chemical-free products from cleaning solutions to napkins to insects (as an alternative to pesticides) for the garden. Most of their products come from Seventh Generation, which has sold environmentally safe household products since 1988. The company's name comes from the Iroquois Confederacy's declaration that, "In our every deliberation, we must consider the impact of our decisions on the next seven generations."

Going organic and vegetarian are private calls. I don't think Ellen will ever go back to her old omnivorous ways, but it's made going to restaurants a challenge. Like it or not, dinner guests can count on lots of leafy greens.

It complicates traveling, too. Ellen and Roger have spent many summers in Maine and cancer wasn't stopping them from beginning to plan their summer pilgrimage. Dealing with the issue in Washington was hard enough—how was she possibly going to address it in Maine?

Roger and I returned that first evening loaded down with grocery bags and in a matter of hours, their kitchen was filled with fresh, wholesome organic bounty. The local health food stores, Fresh Fields and Cash Grocer, had a devoted new customer and Ellen, soothed by soy milk, containers of white tofu, organically-grown bananas and boxes of pesticide-free Kashi, could now eat as well as sleep.

The Apothecary (http://www.intr.net/apothecary)
The Organic Kitchen (http://www.organickitchen.com)
Yahoo!'s organic food page
    (http://dir.yahoo.com/Business_and_Economy/Companies/Food/Natural_Organic)
The Green Marketplace (http://www.greenmarketplace.com)

"In our every deliberation, we must consider the impact of our decisions on the next seven generations."

Giving Up Your Hair

Ellen's hair was silky black. It fell just below her shoulders and swung. Ellen worried Stafford wouldn't recognize her without hair since Stafford had developed the habit of holding onto it like an apron string when she nursed.

Ellen and I come from a world in which people with cancer wear wigs—and you can never tell, but...Wigs? To us, wigs were sort of like girdles—a deployable feminine tool but somehow unworkable and somewhat untenable. They belonged to another time and place, until the prospect of baldness forced us to consider them.

You can get wigs over the Internet via *Studio International,* "The World's Largest On-Line Salon." They offer Cheryl Tiegs wigs, Raquel Welch wigs, human hair wigs, Dolly Parton wigs and wigs cut to look however you want. If you send them a lock of hair, they can match the color. Their Website even features piano music.

Upon reflection, Ellen still couldn't bear to wear a wig.

A friend of her mother's sent some turbans. She thought they made her look like someone with cancer—the way a wig would make her feel. Over the years, Ellen had developed a unique fashion statement involving cowboy boots, long skirts or dresses, tee shirts and scarves wrapped around her neck. When she knew she was going to lose her hair but before it actually fell out, she decided that when the time came, she would simply adapt the neck scarf to her head—cool-girl style.

Ellen also made a hair appointment with Fernando, a hair stylist who had been suggested to her by Carole O'Toole, an ibc survivor. My hair is often short, but, choosing short hair is one thing. Arranging to have your long hair cut to avoid the odd shock of watching it slither down the shower drain is quite another. Her mother and I went to the appointment with her.

Fernando, neither tall nor acutely trim, sat Ellen down in his chair, draped a sheet over her, and spun her around in dizzying circles while, hmmm-hmmming to himself and pulling his chin, he squinted at her. He turned her around so she faced the mirror and proceeded to lop her silky black hair off from behind.

I alternated between stuffing handfuls of it into plastic bags so Stafford would be able to see how gorgeous her mother's hair had been to snapping pictures of the important process.

To us, wigs were sort of like girdles — a deployable feminine tool but somehow unworkable and somewhat untenable.

Snip by snip, Ellen's new look began to emerge. At first it wasn't clear which way it was going to go and she bit her bottom lip as her mother chit-chatted about the various things one could do to look feminine. Fernando raced on. He spun her away from the mirror and worked around her face. She shut her eyes and blew away the remnants. He spun her back to the mirror. I feared she would feel defrocked. She opened her eyes. She looked hot and fashionable and breezy and strong—and, I thought, she knew it. Her whole face glittered with confident delight.

Several days later, much of that hair cut went down the drain. Of the experience, Ellen wrote:

"It came off in the shower in clumps. Then I got out of the shower, tipped over my head and shook it and it fell to the ground in a big heap. Roger was complaining about being late for work. I told him he was going to have to be late and look after Stafford while I cleaned up my hair. I reminded him that this was not a normal morning, that my hair had just come out and that these things were going to happen, but they weren't necessarily all bad—it is just that we were going to have to deal with them."

The rest wound up on her pillow the following morning. That's when the scarves began making their appearance. Around this time, my friend F.K. came to visit me in Washington and the three of us went hat hunting. He suggested the soft caps bike riders sometimes wear beneath their helmets. Ellen loved the idea. Her sister began knitting hats for her. She wore all these things through the winter months and grew increasingly at ease with wearing no hat at all.

She looks quite beautiful without hair, and so feminine that I got mine cut short again, although that didn't work quite as well.

And Stafford? Hair or no hair, that girl knows her mother.

Studio International (http://studiohair.net)

And Stafford? Hair or no hair, that girl knows her mother.

Becoming Acquainted with Survivors

One of the struggles Ellen and I shared revolved around questions of conventionality versus the illusive call to "follow your heart" that rings in the minds of all dreamers.

Back in the dark ages—when my mother was sick—there were two clear paths to follow if you had cancer: conventional treatment—chemotherapy, radiation, and surgery—and unconventional treatment, which covered everything else. My mother pursued conventional treatment until it was, perhaps, too late. She then went to Livingston Wheeler Treatment Center in California, where they advised her, among other things, to eat beans and grains and to visualize her cancer dissolving. Four months later, she died.

Ellen has gracefully and masterfully employed both strategies—a road neither she nor I had ever seen taken first hand, and also one that is not only more common these days, but is also often advised, even by conventional oncologists. Ellen doesn't much care whether she likes beans or not. She eats them, regularly. Because of her open mind and steadfast will to live, Ellen has created her own treatment plan.

Ellen couldn't have developed her treatment plan as quickly or as fully as she did without the help of an angel on earth, Carole O'Toole, who had been diagnosed with ibc in 1993 and survived. Dr. Katherine Alley, the surgeon who performed Ellen's biopsy, put the two in touch.

I went with Ellen to meet Carole, who lives in the Washington area. From the moment Ellen looked at Carole, Ellen was changed. Right then Ellen became, in addition to my peer, my teacher. She and Carole shared something beyond the fact that they had both been required to look at their own deaths at an inopportune time. They shared a unique relationship to life and I knew Ellen would teach me what she could. On a practical level, Carole put Ellen in touch with the people and practices that had helped her live through cancer.

After meeting with Irv Rosenberg, Ellen started biofeedback. She joined a group therapy meeting that included members with life-threatening illnesses and others who had nothing more than ingrown toenails. She did it because she'd read that merely giving and sharing helps promote living. She started talking with the same spiritual advisor Carole talks to. That advisor has helped walk Ellen through each of the hard decisions she has had to make, and has helped her sort out the frightening, complicated emotional aspects of her disease. She began painting a mural on the dining room wall.

Because of her open mind and steadfast will to live, Ellen has created her own treatment plan.

"I'm doing everything I've always been interested in doing," Ellen said after the program was underway. "In a way, I feel so selfish."

Talking with a survivor changed the course of Ellen's life. Ask the oncologist for the name of someone who has lived through it. Call that person. Accept help.

If the doctor doesn't have a survivor's name to give you, try the *Cancer Hope Network*, founded in 1981 as CHEMOcare. Here, a cancer patient is put into online or phone contact with a trained volunteer who survived a similar diagnosis. "Get beyond the diagnosis. Talk to someone who's been there," is one of the Network's slogans.

Thanks to Carole, thanks to cancer, thanks to all of the people contributing to Ellen's life, she is now following her heart.

Cancer Hope Network (http://www.cancerhopenetwork.org)

> *Ask the oncologist for the name of someone who has lived through it. Call that person. Accept help.*

Finding Alternative Treatments Online

You would think a man like Dr. William R. Fair, former head and chair of the Department of Urologic Oncology at Memorial Sloan-Kettering Cancer Center, one of the foremost cancer hospitals in the country, would have some of the most respected, presumably effective doctors treating him for his own colon cancer. Wouldn't you?

After a year of chemotherapy and several surgeries and then a recurrence, Fair's doctor told him a little more chemo might help. Then again it might not. Fair declined. The doctor told him he was making a big mistake. Two years later, that same doctor called Fair to find what in the world he was doing—because Fair was doing just fine.

Fair believes his ongoing life results from the conventional treatments he had, as well as from complementary medicine—nutrition, herbal remedies, yoga, meditation and his own open mind.

In fact, Fair left Memorial Sloan-Kettering to be the chairman of the Clinical Advisory Board for Hælth, LLC. A three-year-old complementary medical center, Hælth addresses chronic illness by combining treatments such as nutritional care, exercise, yoga and traditional Chinese medicine with more conventional treatments. The unusual spelling is actually Anglo-Saxon, the fused 'æ' being a ligature —literally a tying together—which represents the blending of the two worlds of medicine. Hælth, busy developing their office and offerings, will begin taking patients in November 2000.

I heard Fair at a lecture series, "Combining Modern Science and Natural Healing," sponsored by the *Center for Mind-Body Medicine* (CMBM) in Washington, D.C. If CMBM could present a conservative guy like Fair who talked in glowing terms about alternative cancer treatments, I decided, it was worth seeing what else they had to offer.

Impeccably-credentialed founder James S. Gordon, M.D., works hard to educate people about the real benefits of employing the mind and the body when confronting disease. To that end, he hosted a Comprehensive Care Conference in 1998 and again in 1999. Speakers included conventionally-minded doctors, such as Robert E. Wittes, Director of the new Division of Cancer Treatment and Diagnosis at the National Cancer Institute, and true pioneers from the world of alternative (also known as complementary) medicine, such as Stanislaw R. Burzynski, M.D., Ph.D.

Conference transcripts—necessary reading for anyone trying to gain a broader understanding of integrated cancer treatment—are online. Find out for yourself what the doctors doing

If CMBM could get a conservative guy like Dr. Fair to talk in glowing terms about alternative cancer treatments, I decided, it was worth seeing what else they had to offer.

the research think about the antioxidant and vitamin-like substance, Coenzyme Q10, touted as an immune system stimulant; the role of nutrition; the benefits of herbal remedies; and the future of chemotherapy and radiation. These transcripts, laden with research findings and new ideas, might well point you toward courses of treatment your own oncologist hasn't heard about or hasn't mentioned.

Ellen was already venturing along the less-traveled path; it was a great relief and reassurance to find others with much more education and experience describing the road ahead.

The CMBM Website offers some good books, some marginally interesting articles that won't change your life, and the opportunity to read those provocative transcripts, which might.

The CMBM site also links to a very interesting site worth plumbing: *Health World Online*. Created by James Strohecker, a self-confessed seeker, and Dave Robertson, something of a seeker but clearly a bottom line kind of guy, HWO is a mix of money and medicine.

Don't be off-put by the heavy emphasis on profiting from the popular boom in alternative health. For example, HWO has a report tailor-made for your specific illness on sale for a terribly steep $350 if you've got cancer; $250 if your disease is not cancer. Those prices and the money-mindedness of the site threaten to undermine its credibility, but if you stay away from Investor Relations, the Business Center, Marketplace, Healthy Travel... there is knowledge to be gained.

Health World's Quick'Ndex is a pretty amazing resource library covering all manner of alternative health concerns. In the Disease Center, you can click on Cancer and go to a page that allows you to investigate an array of treatment options. Most of the write-ups come from the pages of published books and those books are offered for sale. Some of the information is out-of-date by cancer treatment standards, but there is still a great deal you can learn about different therapies.

Browse around Health World when you have time to sift the good from the not so good. The site is so big it can be hard to navigate if you're in a panicky frame of mind, but if you can calm down and have time to poke around, you may be smarter by the time you leave.

As for the CMBM site, go there no matter what because you will be in the presence of some of the most respected voices in the field.

The Center for Mind-Body Medicine (http://www.cmbm.org)
Health World Online (http://ww.healthy.net/welcome/index.asp)

... go there no matter what because you will be in the presence of some of the most respected voices in the field.

Checking Out The Non-Conventional

Alternative medicine. Complementary medicine. You say tomato. I say tomato. "Alternative" acquired such a bad name in some circles, the establishment now calls such methods, strategies and practices "complementary" medicine.

No matter what you call it, half the cancer patients in the United States seek out some form of non-conventional treatment. They spend an estimated $13 billion annually, according to the Center for Alternative Medicine Research at the University of Texas-Houston, one of the 11 Specialty Research Centers funded by the *National Center for Complementary and Alternative Medicine*, (NCCAM.)

Ellen does not drink Essiac tea, a popular herbal remedy whose principal ingredients are burdock root, Indian rhubarb, sheep sorrel, and slippery elm, but she might if someone gave her some. Perhaps she is crazy to take all the supplements she does take. She is certainly not foregoing chemotherapy. She's had surgery—during which her surgeon read a prayer Ellen had written. She'll have radiation, too, although radiation for Hodgkin's is what some oncologists think caused her breast cancer in the first place. Without doubt, she's following the conventional treatment plan.

Many people turn to complementary medicine late in what becomes a fight with cancer. If it doesn't work, the outfit providing the complementary medicine is often perceived to have been fraudulent. My mother turned to alternative medicine late in the game. It did not work. I don't think the clinic, where she received alternative treatment, was or is fraudulent. Maybe it could have worked had my mother gone earlier. I don't know.

At the same time, there are some "alternative practitioners" who probably are fraudulent. This is terribly uncertain territory and you will simply have to decide for yourself.

There are scores of places on the Internet where you can learn about complementary medicine. A good place to test the waters is NCCAM, established by Congressional mandate in 1998 to conduct and support research and training, and spread information. Their site—which lists research funding opportunities for scientists who want to do research on alternative therapies that offer promise for the future—is similar to other government sites—awash with words, but thin on realistically useful, practical information for people who need help here and now.

NCCAM funds 11 Specialty Research Centers which "study complementary and alternative

> *... half the cancer patients in the United States seek out some form of nonconventional treatment. They spend an estimated $13 billion annually...*

treatments for specific health conditions." As designated by NCCAM, the University of Texas Health Science Center studies alternative and complementary treatments for cancer.

The University of Texas's Center for Alternative Medicine Research in Cancer (UTCAM) presents the progeny of a very workable marriage between different disciplines—conventional and unconventional—that do not need to be in opposition, but so often are.

UTCAM's Webpage is easy on the eyes. It is appealing to read about alternative medicine in relatively dry language stripped of the hyperbole or scorn-for-convention that so often accompanies discussions of complementary medicine. You can access long thorough critiques of the therapies UTCAM is studying. You can read about the investigators and their scientific and clinical staff. You can send emails if you want to.

For anyone who does not want to be preyed upon in a moment of desperation but longs for information, this is an excellent place to start looking. You will see what is being hawked on the alternative market, and you may see something you like—backed up by science you trust.

At the same time, no discussion of alternative medicine on the Web is complete without the inclusion of Dr. Stephen Barrett's site, *Quackwatch*. Quackwatch lambastes and condemns every alternative strategy I've ever heard mentioned. I think Dr. Barrett is an overzealous antagonist, but he is thorough and committed to his viewpoint.

Seeing both sides of the story can only help.

National Center for Complementary and Alternative Medicine (NCCAM)
    (http://nccam.nih.gov)
The University of Texas's Center for Alternative Medicine Research in Cancer (UTCAM)
    (http://www.sph.uth.tmc.edu/utcam)
Quackwatch (http://www.quackwatch.com)

For anyone who does not want to be preyed upon in a moment of desperation but longs for information, this is an excellent place to start looking.

Keeping on Top of the News

Researching for this book has been like writing letters to Ellen. It has kept her foremost in my mind. Reading, thinking, and writing about cancer has given me a way—even a small way—to help. Providing these services is how I have expressed my grief and offered my prayers for her.

I talked with my brother, Ted, recently. He and his wife, Jenny, argue over the amount of time he spends with a friend whose wife has breast cancer. Jenny thinks Ted is ignoring their family. Ted remembers what it felt like when our mother got sick.

Perhaps, my brother and I are trying to recapture our freshest memories of what the world felt like when our mother was here. Maybe we are repaying a debt to those who helped us as we struggled through her illness. Maybe we are doing what we can to make sure those we care about feel as grounded and as safe as possible, when their world is exploding in incomprehensible ways.

Whatever it is, it turned me into an activist, eager to jump in and research every possibility at the slightest sign that Ellen might be served. So, when she mentioned that she had heard something about breast milk neutralizing cancer cells, I went to work. I checked into the national breast cancer conversation to see what I could find.

I visited *The Washington Post* Website and went to the health section where I found overviews and broad-brush-stroke information about breast cancer. Given a choice, I'd depend on OncoLink or another medical institution for medical information. Stories at The Post only 14 days old are free—scroll to the bottom of the home page and on the right hand side, where it says, "Search the Post," and type in breast cancer. I found 24 stories of varying usefulness—but some were good. Unfortunately, if you want to read most archived articles—click Archives on the Webpage and type in Breast Cancer—the Post charges between $1.50 and $2.50. The upside is that you can compile a list of want-to-reads and truck to the library knowing exactly where to go in the microfiche.

All current articles at *The New York Times* are free on the Web, but you have to register, as you will find out once you ask to see anything besides the front page of the day's paper. Registering is painless. Most archived articles cost $2.50, though some are free. To see if the paper has anything you want, click Archive on the front page and type in the term or terms you want.

Most other major papers operate the same way—the day's news and select articles are free

> *Maybe we are doing what we can to make sure those we care about feel as grounded and as safe as possible, when their world is exploding in incomprehensible ways.*

while most archived pieces cost—but it never hurts to be armed with addresses: The Los Angeles Times, The Miami Herald, The Chicago Tribune, and The Boston Globe—they are all online.

There is a full list of all online newspapers at the *American Journalism Review's Newslink*. Searching each paper for Breast Cancer will cough up a few things, perhaps useful, that won't cost money.

USA TODAY is a different story. You can search their archives back to 1987—no charge. USA TODAY also has a cancer page with articles on the day's issues and ideas, many written by Associated Press reporters.

If you can afford it, *The Electric Library* is a shortcut that lets you search major newspapers (including USA TODAY), radio, television and government transcripts as well as an astonishing number of good magazines, newswires and books. You can get a free 30-day trial membership to see if you like it, then subscribe for $9.95 a month or $59.95 a year.

As for television sources online, *MSNBC's* breast cancer page is packed with well-presented, easily accessible information. *CNN* has a page dedicated to women's health, too, but for the best cancer-related articles, go straight to the page they use to feature cancer-related articles.

This may seem like too many addresses until you get going. You'll have to pick and choose, but it's straightforward and non-taxing. While I didn't find anything saying breast milk neutralized cancer cells, I was soon familiar with the most talked about cancer-related issues of the day. I was also now much better prepared for the next excursion onto the Web in search of specific topics. More importantly, I got to spend a day doing something worthwhile for someone whose life was, to me, worth keeping. And I realized how lucky I have been, for Ellen has allowed me to help.

The Washington Post (http://www.washingtonpost.com)
The New York Times (http://www.nytimes.com)
American Journalism Review Newslink (http://ajr.newslink.org/menu.html)
USA TODAY (http://www.usatoday.com)
The Electric Library (http://www.elibrary.com)
MSNBC breast cancer page (http://www.msnbc.com/news/BRCANCER_Front.asp)
CNN women's health page (http://cnn.com/HEALTH/indepth.health/womens.health/index.html)

I was soon familiar with the most talked about cancer-related issues of the day.

VISIT US ONLINE @ FIRSTAIDYOURSELF.ORG

Staying Informed for Free

Cancer is expensive. Insurance covers a lot of the costs, but there will always be things you want that insurance doesn't even know how to spell. Sound nutritional advice, for example, is covered by some insurance companies but not by others. As for organic groceries—some people will want this and some will not—no one's insurance company is going to give this request the time of day.

Most anyone whose spouse or child or parent or sibling gets cancer is going to be acutely aware of the coming financial burdens. They may keep their worries to themselves, and quietly liquidate assets to shore up the bank account or they may groan about the costs on the near horizon. Either way, it's going to occur to everyone.

During some of Ellen's most grueling times, Roger visibly applied himself to paying the enormous bills. For the most part, he kept the money worries to himself. He didn't say boo about the biofeedback. I don't think he mentioned the hundreds of dollars worth of vitamins Ellen bought and consumed each month. He wasn't fazed by the expense of her trips back and forth to Sloan-Kettering to see her doctors. He overlooked the high price of organic foods and didn't bat a lash when other foods were thrown out.

He did mention the water—bottled water was expensive. I wanted to shoot him for that but, when I realized he wasn't going to restrict Ellen to tap water, the feeling passed.

Thankfully (or not) having cancer is also sort of like joining a club. Some members are more educated than others and some realize just how dear time and money can be when a diagnosis of cancer comes down. These people, saviors of a kind, give freely. Earlier, I mentioned cancer survivors who did this. Right now it's time to mention some of the people who provide necessary news—free.

Richard K. J. Brown, M.D., board-certified in the fields of Nuclear Medicine and Diagnostic Radiology is such a man. Having worked extensively with oncology patients, he developed *Cancer News*.

The site itself is extensive, well-tended, and easy to use. The information is current and produced by credible sources—although that does not mean their answers are necessarily the right ones for you. There are some links to links to ever more links, and that can finally feel

Most anyone whose spouse or child or parent or sibling gets cancer is going to be acutely aware of the coming financial burdens.

50

An Original WebPointers™ Interactive Internet Guide © 2000 Hope Springs Press Inc

labyrinthine and pointless, but there are also plenty of links that take you directly to the information you are seeking.

If you are still lacking the information you need, and don't have time to sift through archives of major newspapers to see what information is affordable and what is not, try *Yahoo!'s breast cancer coverage* address. When I last checked, the Yahoo News Site offered 10 current and relevant articles from the likes of the BBC, Boston Globe, and Reuters. Free.

There's even more at *NewsEdge/NewsPage*, a serious entrepreneurial venture making the most of our need for minute-to-minute news. NewsPage combs through more than 40 sources each day and posts what they deem noteworthy. On the top right hand corner of the home page, key in Breast Cancer to see what's available. I never found anything of crucial importance, but did stumble across a heads-up about the Comprehensive Cancer Conference II, sponsored by the Center for Mind-Body Medicine and the National Cancer Institute. No other news source I looked at mentioned it.

I was constantly inspired by the generosity of the people and organizations who had chosen to give so freely of their knowledge. They gave me a way to transform my own contribution of time into something really useful.

Cancer News (http://cancernews.com/quickload.htm)
Yahoo breast cancer coverage (http://headlines.yahoo.com/Full_Coverage/Tech/Breast_Cancer)
NewsEdge/NewsPage (www.newspage.com)

If you are still lacking the information you need ... try Yahoo!'s breast cancer coverage address.

Coping with Costs

Stafford was born only seven months before Ellen's diagnosis. Anticipating her arrival, Ellen and Roger boosted their insurance coverage. This stealthy influence from an unborn child represents one more way in which Stafford helped save her mother's life—great insurance allowed for great treatment. Not everyone is so lucky.

The costs of cancer, a catastrophic illness, can be catastrophic as well. It would not be right to say money is tight in the Grayson family, but it is correct to say it is watched, as it is in most every family. So very much of it was going out after Ellen got sick that what remained was watched very closely indeed.

No matter what your circumstances, when cancer strikes money becomes a concern and the insurance company is going to play a major role in how big a concern it becomes.

Virginia Hetrick's *You Are Not Alone* (YANA), has excellent, easy-to-read, incredibly helpful pages about *keeping medical records*. Everything from "Basic Information About Yourself. . ." to "Legal Paperwork" and "Receipts" is covered.

If you're working with Medicare, Medicaid or the Child Health Insurance Program, you can use the Webpage for the *Health Care Financing Administration* (HCFA). The site is not enormously helpful, but click on the category of interest in the left-hand column boxes and you'll be taken to pages with information.

There is also a single address you can use to get relevant *HCFA phone numbers* if that's what you need. Depending on which category you choose, you'll get an offering of "800" numbers as well as numbers to state contacts, state insurance commissioner's offices, regional official offices, and federal contacts.

If you're having trouble getting claims processed or even understanding your insurance company's rules, spend some time at the *Cancer Care* site. This nonprofit organization provides a myriad of services to cancer patients, including helping with certain costs. Executive Director Diane S. Blum was a social work supervisor at Memorial Sloan-Kettering Cancer Center and at Dana Farber Cancer Institute before joining Cancer Care.

Cancer Care has very good targeted articles on aspects of insurance problems that may arise. Examples of topics addressed are "*HMO's and Other Managed Care Plans,*" "*Information

The costs of cancer, a catastrophic illness, can be catastrophic as well.

about 1986 COBRA Plans," "Medical Insurance—a 'Hidden Crisis' for a Growing Number of Cancer Patients," and "Getting the Most Our of Your Health Insurance."

Another good place to look for general information and for actual help if you live in New York, New Jersey, Pennsylvania, Connecticut, or Texas is the nonprofit organization *Health Care Choices*. Click on "Health Insurance Resources Center." Their goal is to educate people about the nation's confusing health care system.

If you've read all there is to read and still have questions and problems, consider the *Patient Advocate Foundation*, a nonprofit organized by Nancy Davenport-Ennis and her husband, John, in memory of Cheryl Grimmel. The Foundation posts relevant articles and bulletins on the Internet and offers legal consulting and referral services for patients involved in an insurance crisis. They not only have a National Legal Resource Network, but also a National Managed Care Resource Network.

Both the site and the Patient Advocate Foundation are godsends.

You Are Not Alone (YANA) keeping medical records (http://www.yana.org/medicalrecords.htm)
Health Care Financing Administration (http://www.hcfa.gov)
HCFA phone numbers (http://www.hcfa.gov/regions/default.htm)
Cancer Care (http://www.cancercareinc.org)
Cancer Care "HMO's and Other Managed Care Plans"
    (http://www.cancercare.org/patients/hmos.htm)
Cancer Care "Information about 1986 COBRA Plans"
    (http://www.cancercare.org/patients/cobra.htm)
Cancer Care "Medical Insurance—a 'Hidden Crisis' for a Growing Number of Cancer Patients"
    (http://www.cancercare.org/patients/crisis.htm)
Cancer Care "Getting the Most Our of Your Health Insurance"
    (http://www.cancercare.org/clinical/insur13.htm)
Health Care Choices (http://www.healthcarechoices.org/contact.htm)
The Patient Advocate Foundation (http://www.patientadvocate.org)

If you've read all there is to read and still have questions and problems, consider the Patient Advocate Foundation...

Sharing and Giving Back

Early March. I was going to be extra hands at Ellen and Roger's for a week. Ellen's hair was long gone and she was getting used to her strict (but modified) vegetarian diet.

Ellen's sister, Page, had been helping Ellen for a week. Ellen's other sister, Pam, had been there earlier. Stafford was teething and made more fretful by the constant turnover.

Page showed me around the kitchen. Then it got serious. "This is how you make Stafford's bottle. She gets eight ounces at 6 a.m., then six ounces at 9:30.... This is how you make her lunch. And *this* is how you hold her." Stafford is my goddaughter. Until then, I had never held a baby long enough to feel competent about it. Stafford and I had some ice to break and I, for one, thought we had to break it fast. Ellen needed a helper—not a misfit.

As the week progressed, Ellen and I did beautifully. Roger and I, unaccustomed to each other in this setting, had our ups and downs. The whole thing was utterly disturbing and disruptive for him. I wanted to keep it from being that way for Ellen. The week had its tough moments.

Every evening, Roger closed the living room doors and listened to blues while I went upstairs, guzzled two beers and wrote in my journal. Or so I said. In reality, I stared at the red light indicator on their telephone that told me Roger was using the phone.

At Ellen and Roger's, I had determined not to be like the babysitter who comes over and prefers the telephone to the baby. My friend F.K. and I usually stayed in close touch via telephone and email but the computer was unavailable and I had asked him not to call me at their house. Ellen might be snoozing, diapers might be getting changed, or some other minor domestic situation might find me too distracted to yap freely. Still, I was desperate to talk to him. Many nights I watched that red light, waiting for the chance to use the phone, a chance that seldom came before I fell asleep, exhausted, grieving for myself.

Outside, the world sparkled from heavy snow fall. One day Ellen and I set out to fetch a prescription and stopped to get stamps for an elegantly-touching response she was sending to approximately 200 people who had written or called with prayers and concern.

Wrapped in coats and gloves and hats, we picked our way through the trodden snow and talked about ways to make ourselves useful in the world while giving back to it.

We shall each find our ways, but that cold afternoon, we talked about designing a retreat—a

As the week progressed, Ellen and I did beautifully. Roger and I, unaccustomed to each other in this setting, had our ups and downs.

retreat offering the best of what Ellen was learning. A place people with and without cancer could learn about biofeedback, yoga, good nutrition, the spiritual or emotional roots of disease and the growth that was possible. We'd call it Starpoint 3, a name that came to Ellen in a dream.

In fact, such a place already exists. The *Commonweal Cancer Help Program* (CCHP), founded by Michael Lerner, is a retreat in Bolinas, California, for people with cancer. It is both a Mecca and an oasis. It is a week of exploration involving deep relaxation, meditation, massage, art, imagery, a vegetarian diet, communion with others in a similar situation and things that defy language. The fee is $1,480 per person. It is not treatment, as we know it.

At the Website you can also read some of the pivotal texts of complementary medicine, including Lerner's "Choices in Healing: Integrating the Best of Conventional and Complementary Approaches to Cancer." The entire Congressional publication, "Unconventional Cancer Treatments," that came from the now-defunct Office of Technology Assessment (OTA) is also available. Lerner contributed to it. Other articles are there as well, in addition to a neatly presented and explained list of links, some of which you can find everywhere else, some of which are unique to this site.

Because of Commonweal's success and popularity—they have a nine-month waiting list—other Commonweal-esque programs have been born around the country.

Walking that day with Ellen, I vaguely recalled Commonweal's existence from the days of my mother's illness. I had read OTA's assessment of alternative treatments then. Later, when I found their Website, building a better mousetrap was out of the question. Commonweal has it all.

Thinking about that mousetrap, however, gave Ellen and me great joy on that bright, cold day as we headed home, shook the snow off our boots and re-entered the world of quiet stormy tension.

That night, my first call to Chicago got no answer. When I'd waited long enough to try again—about seven seconds, the red busy light was already glowing. Lonely and frustrated, I wrote in my journal, sure that F.K. would understand.

That day, his mother was diagnosed with lung cancer.

Cancer is impossible to explain if you haven't been there. Now F.K. was there too.

Commonweal (http://www.commonweal.org)

Cancer is impossible to explain if you haven't been there. Now F.K. was there too.

Finding Other Retreats

For a long time, Ellen considered visiting a retreat. Had she ultimately wished to do so, she could have found programs in the east that replicated the Commonweal experience. Because she was already investigating many of the opportunities such retreats offered, she chose instead to visit a monastery in Virginia. What she really needed, she decided, was unscheduled time—alone.

Not everyone is in a position to cobble together a personal complementary treatment package without leaving their area, and luckily there are some excellent options available.

The Commonweal program is so popular, however, that there is a long waiting list. Yet, there is such desire and need for its special blend of support and inspiration that a handful of independent organizations have sprung up to help meet the demand. Each of the retreats mentioned in this chapter was inspired by Commonweal and Commonweal has been involved with them either through training, consultation or both.

Two of the organizations—*Smith Farm Cancer Help Program* and the *Ting-Sha Institute*—are closely tied to Commonweal.

Smith Farm, in Washington, D.C., is an east coast version of Commonweal, and was co-founded by Barbara Smith Coleman, a Washington-based artist and cancer survivor, and Michael Lerner, who serves as president of both institutions.

Smith Farm's headquarters are in Georgetown and their residential retreats are located in surrounding rural areas. That is where the most intense exploration of the healing arts and sciences—yoga, deep relaxation, meditation, massage—takes place. Participants must be under the care of a doctor and must be able to tend to their own needs. Dr. Rachel Naomi Remen, M.D., author of "Kitchen Table Wisdom: Stories that Heal," and a leader at Commonweal, frequently leads educational discussions at Smith Farm.

Another Commonweal collaboration, Ting-Sha Institute in Point Reyes, California, was founded in 1972 and offers a series of cancer retreats throughout the year. One of its founding principles is to "[d]emonstrate that activities which are conventionally described as medicine, art, psychotherapy and spiritual practices are not isolated from each other." Their cancer program, which in

... there is such desire and need for its special blend of support and inspiration that a handful of independent organizations have sprung up to help meet the demand.

1999 cost $1550 per person for a week's retreat, reflects that understanding. The director, Virginia Veach, is a founding staff member of the Cancer Help Program at Commonweal.

Harmony Hill in Union, Washington, offers cancer retreats as well. Their focus is healing through "becoming whole emotionally, mentally, and spiritually." Retreats are limited to eight people. Gretchen Schodde, executive director of Harmony Hill, founded the retreat in 1986.

The Callanish Healing Retreats Society, located in Vancouver, British Columbia, was inspired by the Commonweal program. In fact, Janie Brown, executive director of Callanish Healing Retreats Society, trained at Commonweal in 1995 and went on to create the first program of this kind in Canada. Callanish offers six week-long retreats during the year. Brown's groups are also limited to eight people.

The Hawaii Cancer Help Retreats, endorsed by Commonweal, apparently has no Website—I couldn't find one, anyway—but can be contacted by calling: 808-885-0995 or 808-885-7547.

The majority of these organizations also offer retreats and educational opportunities for health care professionals who work with those with terminal illnesses.

Smith Farm Center for the Healing Arts (http://www.smithfarm.com)
Ting-Sha Cancer Help Program (http://www.amacord.com/tingsha/index.html)
Harmony Hill (http://www.harmonyhill.org)
The Callanish Healing Retreats Society (http://www.callanish.org)

Their focus is healing through "becoming whole emotionally, mentally, and spiritually."

Remembering to Take Care of Yourself

If you're reading this, you are probably close to someone who has cancer. You may be lending a significant hand. This makes you a caregiver. I don't like the word, but the role is privileged.

Whatever you call it, it is also demanding. You can get exhausted, yet you feel guilty thinking of your own routine discomfort. You feel like biting people who don't understand. A sick person is forced to accept help and loving kindness, willy-nilly. A well caregiver can still pretend to be in control—except that he or she can't take away the illness or the pain.

People will say to you, "Don't forget to take care of yourself." What do they mean? Keep your nails clipped? Go for a pretty drive?

After the first tough week staying at Roger and Ellen's, things only got worse. Now F.K.'s mother had lung cancer. I knew how to pitch in when my mother was sick. I had some ideas when Ellen got sick. But I had no idea what it meant when it happened to the mother of someone I loved, especially when I loved that mother, whom I had known my whole life, as well. I was baffled.

I waited for a signal from F.K. A few days after his mother's cancer was diagnosed, he invited me to Chicago. From there, we went to our hometown and spent the weekend with his family. I felt a little uncomfortable being there at such an intensely personal time, but there I was and glad for it. Then F.K. told me his work demands had increased—he would be going to Europe for almost two weeks out of every month. I was too overwhelmed myself to fully understand the pressure that was building up for him.

Back in Washington, Roger and Ellen and I set up a schedule that had me spending several nights with them and going to Sloan-Kettering in New York with Ellen. As we planned the schedule, Roger joked "Oh yes, and I guess Betsy will need a little time to visit F.K." This made me furious because too little existed. Later, Ellen would have additional help, but not yet. I had no idea what F.K. wanted or needed from me. I longed for more time.

The first test of our attachment proved more rigorous than I'd ever imagined. I made decisions based on what I thought I would best be able to live with, given all possible outcomes. It was very difficult. Deep in my heart, I thought he and I would find some path, no matter how rocky, through the wrenching realities and outlandish timing. But something seemed off between us. Or maybe it was my imagination. I was wrapped so tightly I couldn't tell.

> *People will say to you, "Don't forget to take care of yourself." What do they mean? Keep your nails clipped? Go for a pretty drive?*

Many who have subordinated their lives to help a friend or family member have similar stories to tell. Certain impossible aspects of "caregiving" repeat themselves. Dealing with the prospect of death is hard enough. Add to that the unavoidable jostles of life and some things become unworkable. I tried to find answers in the ceiling at night. The Internet offers other solutions.

Y-ME National Breast Cancer Organization, created in 1978 by two survivors, has information for anyone affected by breast cancer—families, friends, children and caregivers. The article, "*When The Woman You Love Has Breast Cancer*," is written for spouses and lovers, but some insights are universal and apply whatever your relationship to the person with cancer.

OncoLink, the University of Pennsylvania's online Cancer Center has two on-target sites. There you'll find a *Caregiver Education Course*. The calm tone suggests everything is fine and normal when really it is neither, but the course is experience-based and you may find it helpful.

OncoLink's "Ten Ways to *Care for the Caregiver*" urges you to take time off.

A Christian group, Cancer Advocate, offers "*A Caregiver's Bill of Rights*," which might resonate. They also offer tips on *Caregiver Burnout*.

None of these sites is world-shaking, but they provide clues about pitfalls that may lie ahead.

Ellen and I returned from New York on a cold, wet Saturday. She'd picked up a bad cold which could be dangerous on top of her chemotherapy. At the house, Roger was laid low by an inner ear disorder that had plagued him for years. Stafford, miserable from her own first cold, needed constant tending. Ellen's mother had been holding down the fort while we were in New York and I spent the night just in case the whole thing blew.

The next day I went to Chicago. F.K. and I were ill-equipped to understand why we could no longer carry on a conversation that made sense to both of us. I caught an early plane home.

Within weeks, he ended the relationship altogether.

Y-ME National Breast Cancer Organization (http://www.yme.org)
When The Woman You Love Has Breast Cancer (http://www.y-me.org/partner.html)
OncoLink's Caregiver Education Course (http://oncolink.upenn.edu/psychosocial/caregivers)
Care for the Caregiver (http://oncolink.upenn.edu/psychosocial/caregivers/care_caregiver.html)
Cancer Advocate's Caregiver's Bill of Rights (http://caregiver.com/rights.html)
Cancer Advocate's Caregiver Burnout (http://caregiver.com/march-april97/articles/burnout.html)

I tried to find answers in the ceiling at night. The Internet offers other solutions.

Paying Attention to Drugs

It was Friday, April 9. Roger, needing a break, went to an antique show in Philadelphia where he planned to spend the night. Besides Ellen and Stafford, antiques are his passion and joy. I, now nursing a wounded heart, planned to spend the night with Ellen. Just in case. Just for comfort. I was glad for her company.

Ellen was in bed. Some days she stayed in her nightgown, but rarely did she retreat to bed. She felt lousy and on top of that, wished Roger was there. She put Stafford to sleep and wanted to ignore her own growing fever. I heated up some chicken stock and read to her while she meekly swallowed one spoonful after another. An hour later, she felt worse. When she finally agreed to go the hospital, around 7:30 p.m., she pulled herself out of bed, threw on two sweaters and a leather jacket, in April, and pale and cold with chemotherapy and cancer, declared that she would drive herself to the emergency room. I fetched a neighbor for Stafford and told Ellen, sweetly, that she was crazy. Without protest, she slid into the passenger's seat.

This emergency room resembled any other on a Friday night. Bloody men, crying children, moaning women. The nurses appeared lethargic about tending to the various emergencies. Eventually they took Ellen away, ran some blood tests and gave her something to bring her fever down; but didn't release her until she broke down in tears of fatigue and frustration near midnight. In the car, she told me her white blood count had been a drastically low 200; doctors don't like to see it fall below 1,000. Four thousand is considered normal.

I'd read up on the chemotherapy drugs she was being given, but missed something crucial—"The lowering of the white blood cells that fight infections is known as *neutropenia*. It is the most important complication of chemotherapy. It is almost always due to impairment of bone marrow to produce cells and... is most severe in patients who receive aggressive treatments ... **if left untreated, this complication may become fatal in a matter of hours.**"

Go to *Tirgan Oncology Associates's* site for a description of neutropenia and read a discussion of other common chemotherapy side effects while you are there. Dr. Tirgan is a board certified medical oncologist who trained at Boston University. Nosing around Tirgan's pages will answer some chemo questions. His Holistic Beauty site has a variety of soothing pictures—birds, flowers, places, light—and if you have time, you might stop in for a pleasant interlude.

... if left untreated, this complication may become fatal in a matter of hours."

The *Internet Drug Index* is a good place to see patient package information inserts for chemotherapeutic agents. In the search box, type in the drug you want to learn about. One I researched was Adriamycin (doxorubicin), one of the chemotherapy agents Ellen was taking. I noticed the instruction to "Call your prescriber or health care professional if you have a fever, chills, sore throat or other symptoms of a cold or flu." Read the fine print. Take the directions and warnings seriously.

CenterWatch provides a list of drugs approved for use in the United States. The P/S/L Consulting Group's *Doctors Guide to the Internet* has a list of drugs approved around the world. It is common to read about an excellent drug being used successfully in another country, but prohibited here. Depending on the direness of the situation, you can always try to get to that other country.

If you'd like manufacturer's press releases or sales figures on chemotherapy drugs, you can find that at the P/S/L Consulting Group's Doctors Guide to the Internet, too. The site is sponsored by many pharmaceutical corporations and who knows—you might scroll into some late-breaking news.

The next morning, Ellen woke up feeling better. Roger pulled in around 11 a.m. and unveiled a chic new Polo outfit—blue shorts, cute cardigan sweater—for Stafford. If he was concerned about Ellen's brush with emergency, the back and forth of casual banter hid it well.

Ellen fingered the sweater's gold buttons.

"Roger," she said, "Stafford isn't going to fit into these for about five years. What are you thinking?"

"She is so," he said, holding the shorts up next to Stafford, who completely disappeared behind them.

Tirgan Oncology Associates (http://www.tirgan.com)
Neutropenia (http://www.tirgan.com/leucpnia.htm)
The Internet Drug Index (http://rxlist.com)
CenterWatch drugs approved for use (http://www.centerwatch.com/drugs/DRUGLIST.HTM)
Doctors Guide to the Internet (http://www.pslgroup.com/docguide.htm)

Read the fine print. Take the directions and warnings seriously.

Paying Attention to Paying

Ellen's unique circumstances allowed her to pursue complementary treatments with vigor. As she delved ever more deeply into them, she was increasingly disturbed that other women—low income women in particular—would not have access, primarily because they couldn't afford it.

The various strategies Ellen embraced—meditation, biofeedback, excellent nutrition, talking with a spiritual advisor, Chinese medicine—can be seen as dilettantish new age pastimes (though I, for one, am a believer in them). Pursuing these avenues can be expensive. Because the results of such strategies are hard to quantify, most insurance policies do not cover their costs.

Although Ellen had always meant to look into these subjects, she didn't explore them until it was time to save her life. Since they have helped her, she reasonably thought they could help other people. But how was a low-income woman with a fresh cancer diagnosis supposed to learn about meditation? And even if she did hear about it as a potential lifesaving tool, how was she going to afford it?

These were the sorts of questions we asked each other as the different treatments progressed. As I looked into ways low-income women could learn about acupuncture and similar therapies, a more fundamental question developed: who is helping low-income women pay for treatments?

Sadly there is not much help, but it does exist.

On the complementary side, the *Charlotte Maxwell Complimentary Clinic* in Oakland, California, represents a bastion of useful concern. Named in memory of Charlotte Maxwell, the clinic is staffed by "a group of health care practitioners and friends of women with cancer who have joined together to make complementary forms of care available to women who ordinarily couldn't afford to pay..." They offer acupuncture, homeopathy, massage, visualization and hypnotherapy—to be taken advantage of in conjunction with treatment overseen by a primary care physician.

As for help funding routine cancer treatment, there are different clinics in different states that rise to the challenge. Drug companies, too, sometimes have reimbursement programs. The *Susan G. Komen Breast Cancer Foundation* also raises money and contributes to programs and clinics around the country that help fund treatment for low-income women. The Komen Foun-

a more fundamental question developed: who is helping low-income women pay for treatments?

dation was founded by Nancy Goodman Brinker in memory of her sister, who died of breast cancer at the age of 36. The best way to hook into what's available in any given state is to call the Susan G. Komen Breast Cancer Foundation (the Race for the Cure people) at 1-800-462-9273. Ask to be connected to Affiliate Services, and explain your situation and needs.

The *California Breast Cancer Treatment Fund* (CBCTF), for example, is a Komen Foundation affiliate. The CBCTF helps cover treatment costs for residents of California who have no insurance and no links to medical services. Comparable Komen affiliates exist in every state.

Cancer Care's financial assistance program provides funds "for needs such as home care, child care, pain medication, and transportation to treatment." They now provide more than $1 million annually in support for eligible residents in Connecticut, New Jersey and New York. The New York Community Trust provides a special fund for the medically indigent.

In Florida, the nonprofit organization *Bosom Buddies Breast Cancer Support, Inc.*, has assistance funds for low-income resident women. In 1998, they disbursed $33,197 to a total of 55 clients.

The only good thing about the scarcity of help for low-income women is that the breast cancer community at-large is aware of this tragedy and so often tragedy paves the way for change.

Charlotte Maxwell Complimentary Clinic (http://www.acupuncture.com/Referrals/Char.htm)
The Susan G. Komen Breast Cancer Foundation (http://www.breastcancerinfo.com)
California Breast Cancer Treatment Fund (http://www.chpscc.org/bcedp/trtmnt.html)
Cancer Care's financial assistance program (http://www.cancercare.org/services/services.htm)
Bosom Buddies Breast Cancer Support, Inc (http://www.go-icons.com/bosombuddies.htm)

... the breast cancer community at-large is aware of this tragedy and so often tragedy paves the way for change.

Finding Help Around the Home

Cancer comes. The house still needs to be cleaned. The baby—fed, entertained, and bathed. Laundry needs to be done. Dinners need to be cooked, often with new and unfamiliar foods. Needs are everywhere.

How are people supposed to do all this while putting their energy into finding doctors, going to appointments, enduring chemo and generally struggling against a life-threatening illness?

Ellen and Roger already had a wonderful Peruvian couple who came every two weeks and cleaned their house. They also had Minnie, taciturn and gentle, who came and watched Stafford from 10 a.m. to 3 p.m. each weekday. Other routine needs of a growing family presented major obstacles.

Although Ellen's sisters came and helped, they both led busy lives in faraway states where each also had a young child and a husband. I was planning to start work when I arrived in my new destination—wherever that was to be, and I wasn't certain—so my days were free. I understood some of the demands of cancer from my experience with my mother, and now Ellen's predicament made my prior routine lose much of its urgency. I chipped in, which meant going to doctors appointments, chemo infusions, sometimes to the grocery store, and fetching new clothes for a growing baby.

Although the arrangement seemed written in the stars, Ellen knew I planned to leave and that to some extent, her situation was keeping me in Washington. While I wanted to be by her side, I also knew it wouldn't work for months on end. For one thing, I couldn't cook. Ellen needed someone to prepare meals for her. When she was receiving monstrously high doses of chemotherapy, food did not appeal to her. Roger couldn't deal with tofu. Ellen simply wasn't up to cooking at all, though she ate as much as she could and so has not wasted away.

She and Roger began giving me money. As grateful as I was, that made me uncomfortable. And the one time I tried to cook, Roger appeared in the kitchen just as I was extinguishing the flaming oven mittens. During one of Ellen's worst experiences with the chemo, she called her mother, who came immediately and continued to come more and more frequently. I still helped, but I could not provide a mother's love—nor her skills in the kitchen.

Around mid-April, Ellen had turned a corner—for the better. Through Ellen's church, her

the one time I tried to cook, Roger appeared in the kitchen just as I was extinguishing the flaming oven mittens.

mother found Priscilla—a young, good, strong woman from the Sudan. I was not at the house when Priscilla first visited for her interview, but the way Ellen and her mother tell it, Priscilla came through the door and brought with her the good light of salvation, solution and hope. She cooked interesting Sudanese recipes using organic foods herself. She loved children, knew exactly how to hold them, and wondered why in this country raising children was not the community and family affair that it was back home. She got on well with Roger. She spoke several languages. Her father was a doctor. She was, by all accounts, perfect.

Ellen and Priscilla grew close. As Priscilla established herself, Ellen told me she knew I had been waiting to leave and if I wished, the time had come. Deeply sad, for that meant good-byes were imminent, and relieved for the same reason, I started focusing on leaving.

Home care is a potential financial burden, but assistance does exist. There are several organizations that can send someone to your house to cook, clean, administer infusions—someone who can help at whatever level is needed. In Canada, the *Victorian Order of Nurses* has taken on this special role.

Cancer Care offers emotional and practical support to cancer patients and others—free of charge. Click on "Immediate Help," and you will quickly see an option: Referrals to Services in your area. There is a phone number, 800-813-HOPE; or scroll down to fill out a referral form on the computer. They also offer a concise Webpage detailing issues worth considering if you use *home care*.

The other place to look is the *National Association for Home Care*. Keying in their address will launch you to a page where you can choose from an array of topical headings, ranging from who pays for home care to a HomeCare & Hospice Locator. Don't let the word "hospice" scare you away. Focus on the Home Care part and get the additional hands you need. It will reduce the stress of the situation and nothing but good can come from that.

Victorian Order of Nurses (http://www.von.ca)
CancerCare (http://www.cancercare.org)
Cancer Care's page on home care (http://www.cancercare.org/hhrd/hhrd_home.htm)
National Association for Home Care (http://www.nahc.org/Consumer/coninfo.html)

Home care is a potential financial burden, but assistance does exist.

Saying Good-byes

Deep spring—late April—found Ellen looking radiant and feeling pretty darned good, though at the time she was still preparing for surgery.

Her doctor at Sloan-Kettering had adjusted her chemotherapy. He explained that his research brainchild, dose-dense chemotherapy, in which the patient receives the highest possible dose of one drug for three weeks running, wasn't working any better or worse than regular doses administered over a longer period of time. He called a halt to her dense doses.

Ellen had not sailed through the high doses, but she tolerated them quite well. Mouth and other sores flattened her a couple of times making the life-sustaining acts of eating and drinking unreasonably hard. She got through it by plying herself with ointments and warm baths and eating and drinking as much as she could. Smaller doses, while not a breeze, promised to be delightfully livable by comparison. She continued the hard work of educating herself about her body, her situation, her God's help and her guides—and her mass continued to shrink.

My first meeting with Priscilla occured when she came one evening as I was attempting to feed Stafford, who was not impressed with her dinner. Minutes after Priscilla arrived, she reached over me, stirred the various dishes of mush I was trying unsuccessfully to sneak into Stafford's mouth, and easily popped in a series of spoonfuls. When bath time came, Stafford rejected Priscilla and accepted me. I was thrilled—and horrified at my raw jealousy. There was no getting around the fact that Priscilla's presence would spell good things for Ellen. I ate my pettiness with Priscilla's wonderful steamy falafel and rich chickpea soup and voluminous salads laced with dandelion and cilantro.

Ellen's health and strength grew visibly. She started looking in catalogues and thinking about bathing suits for her summer in Maine. She learned how to use her computer more efficiently which meant I would no longer be necessary as a middle man when she needed help. She had more energy and time for Stafford. She learned to cook tasty and exotic things. She picked up her paint brushes and continued painting the mural on the dining room wall. She wrote me a note saying, "Betsy... your work here is done—in all the best ways. You got me to where I am right now which, if not out of the woods, is at least to a clearing with solid foundations of hope and means of coping spread out before me."

Victory salted the air, and no matter how many times I'd heard people talk about how hard it

You got me to where I am right now which, if not out of the woods, is at least to a clearing with solid foundations of hope ...

was to let go, it never made an impression until I had to do it myself. It made us both sad, but we both knew the time for me to leave had come. A friend of mine offered to take responsibility for making sure my house was properly sublet, so I was free to go. I started poring over maps and found a westward route.

I accompanied Ellen to one more Wednesday chemo infusion and the following Saturday, went to the local farmers market with Ellen, her mother, and Stafford, who was pulled along in a big, colorful, plastic wagon. Ellen radiated health and wisdom. People practically stopped her in the street to ask her what her secret was.

We had a warm sunny morning. Townsfolk bartered pleasantly with farmers. Ellen and her mother stuffed armfuls of bright flowers into the wagon with Stafford. Next went in brown paper bags of green beans, musty carrots, sweet pea pods and fresh herbs. Stafford's head bobbed contentedly in a sea of bright goodness.

I pulled the wagon loaded with life back to the house, but instead of going inside, we loitered on the sidewalk near my car. They wished me luck and Godspeed and then we draped our arms around each other, put our heads together, and Ellen and her mother promised they would be fine.

Two weeks later, as we all knew, Ellen would lose her breast.

Ellen radiated health and wisdom. People practically stopped her in the street to ask her what her secret was.

Getting a New Breast—or Not

Ellen approached the various challenges of her disease on an as-needed basis, so a couple of months before her mastectomy, she started thinking about whether she wanted a new breast.

Would she feel lopsided with just one? Would her feminine self-image weather the loss of what our culture perceives to be one of womanhood's most prized possessions? Would it be weird to have a breast built onto her chest? Was it exciting to consider the possibilities?

Ultimately, Ellen knew that reconstruction was out of the question for her.

When we were at Sloan-Kettering meeting with famed breast surgeon *Dr. Jeanne A. Petrek* the subject of reconstruction came up. Dr. Petrek told Ellen her mass was still too big to operate on and confirmed what Ellen already knew: that Ellen's body was struggling with high doses of chemotherapy, fighting cancer and recovering from pregnancy. Soon it would also be healing from the mastectomy surgery. With all that stress, all the doctors advocated avoiding further burdening her body with another surgical procedure.

If she was disappointed, she never said so. She absorbed the information with the same equanimity she used to absorb so many other pieces of hard news.

Once you have lost a breast, there are several ways of having a new one, and a permanent one, established. Discussions of new breasts refer to the "breast mound"—a disconcertingly objective way to think of one's breast.

The kind of cancer and the extent of surgery will ultimately dictate the range of available choices, but this is the current run-down: tissue expansion with saline water; a silicone gel implant; flap reconstruction using tissue from the back, lower abdomen, buttocks, or lateral hip area; a latissimus dorsi flap using a specific muscle; a transverse rectus abdominis myocutaneous (TRAM) flap using other specific muscles; and, free flaps using tissue from other places on the body.

The *University of Iowa's Plastic Surgery Webpage* has a fairly technical explanation of these options. There is also a general discussion about when reconstruction ought to be done. The timing depends upon what sort of breast surgery was previously performed.

The *University of Chicago Breast Cancer Comprehensive Center* offers a briefer, less technical discussion of the same topics.

... she wanted a new breast, not just something to stuff into a secret pocket in her bra.

To read about all of this in great depth, try the extraordinarily good *OncoLink* site. You will see pictures here—results of certain procedures—so be prepared.

Bosom Buddies, Inc., an organization created by breast cancer survivors in Florida, sells a $29.95 video about reconstruction. If visuals will help, you can learn more about ordering the video at their Website.

Most of the listed sites seem to be written for doctors. They are chilly.

Patrick Hudson, MDPA, FACS board certified Plastic Surgeon, has a Webpage that is quite patient-friendly. It also doubles as an advertisement for his services, but he makes it easy to read about breast reconstruction. Don't be overly influenced by the graphic of a pink ribbon on his Webpage; they can be downloaded by anyone and do not necessarily represent an official endorsement by an advocacy organization. I know nothing about him except what it says on his Webpage.

After surgery, Ellen found it much easier to view her scar from above than in a full-length mirror. This is when Roger confided to her that her scar was "... kind of neat, as in cool."

About a week after the drainage tubes came out, Ellen went to buy new bras. The sales women at Nordstrom's were wonderful to her and she came home with an array of fancy new gear outfitted with pockets for her prosthesis.

"You know what I've decided?" she said after all this. "I've looked at my chest a lot by now and you know what? It looks like it's winking."

Dr. Jeanne A. Petrek (http://www.mskcc.org/document/CN990610.htm)
University of Iowa Plastic Surgery page
    (http://www.surgery.uiowa.edu:80/surgery/plastic/brecon.html)
University of Chicago Breast Cancer Comprehensive Center
    (http://phoenicia.bsd.uchicago.edu/index.cgi/175005883)
OncoLink (http://www.oncolink.upenn.edu/disease/breast/treat/breast_recon2.html)
Bosom Buddies, Inc (http://www.bosombuddies.org)
Patrick Hudson (http://www.phudson.com/breastrecon.html)

"I've looked at my chest a lot by now and you know what? It looks like it's winking at me."

Flying with the Angels

Ellen has had a couple of important goals besides the major one of getting through this whole ordeal. She wanted to keep the disruption to Stafford's life at a minimum and she didn't want cancer to define her entire life. Both related to relocation and both were remedied by frequent transportation.

Prior to the onset of her cancer, Ellen and Stafford and Roger had been bonding quite nicely. The November before her ibc diagnosis, Ellen left me a phone message saying, "There is poetry going on in this house."

As a result of the cancer, Stafford had to get used to a string of new faces that came and went. Fortunate circumstances allowed Ellen to stay in Washington while visiting her primary oncologist in New York, so the period of changing faces had been relatively short-lived. Mama has usually been home.

She achieved her other goal, too. Since she has been able to fly back and forth when necessary, Ellen has maintained her friendships at home and has kept in close touch with her professional and artistic contacts.

Maintaining stability and staying near home are not startling goals, but not everyone can afford them without outside help. Transportation costs can frequently force patients to forego the best treatment or to uproot career and family in pursuit of that treatment. Fortunately there is outside help for those cancer patients who qualify.

Several groups exist regionally and some nationally which will fly qualifying cancer patients back and forth for medical treatments, consultations and checkups. In most instances, the patient needs to be ambulatory, requiring no form of life support or medical help, and certain financial preconditions must apply, i.e., they must be able to prove financial hardship or need.

One organization will fly patients regardless of their financial resources: *Corporate Angel Network*, headquartered in White Plains, New York. (To become a corporate sponsor at no cost to the corporation, call: 914-328-1313.) Through the Corporate Angel Network (CAN), patients use empty seats on corporate aircraft as they shuttle busy executives between major cities.

CAN is not alone out there. There's an entire subculture of pilots and airlines volunteering their time and service to transporting patients. The *Air Care Alliance* (ACA) has a long list arranged alphabetically, nationally and then regionally. Canada is included. For details on any group,

The November before her ibc diagnosis, Ellen left me a phone message saying, "There is poetry going on in this house."

click on that group's name and you will be taken to its phone number and address. Often there are links to Webpages.

As you'll see, not all the groups fly patients for free. Wings of Freedom tries to find reduced-price tickets for patients; the Emergency Volunteer Aircorps responds to disasters and emergencies... but if you poke around, you'll find that many of these organizations do fly patients to treatment.

To see another long list of charitable flying organizations, go to the National Patient Air Transport Helpline. There are duplicates between these two lists, but each one also has a few the other does not.

The *National Patient Air Transport Helpline* (NPATH) is affiliated with the National Charitable Patient Air Transportation System (NCPATS), which is affiliated with Mercy Medical Airlift Charitable Air Transportation (MMA), which is affiliated with the Air Care Alliance (ACA), founded by Bill Worden in 1990.

Pinning the precise relationships down is probably unimportant. Understanding the services and requirements is not. Most groups do not fly patients if the flight can be covered by insurance or some other means. The guiding mission of the major umbrella groups is to give indigent, low-income or financially vulnerable patients access to distant treatment or to distant facilities for care. All the groups and organizations share the twin roots of compassion and community service.

Luckily for cancer patients, pilots are making poetry in the skies.

Corporate Angel Network (http://www.corpangelnetwork.org)
Air Care Alliance (http://www.aircareall.org/listings.htm)
The National Patient Air Transport Helpline (http://www.npath.org/index.a.html)

All the groups and organizations share the twin roots of compassion and community service.

Losing and Regaining a Breast

Upon learning of the cancer, Ellen did not feel favorably towards her breast. It had let her down, it was diseased and she wanted it taken off. This sounded like a typical reaction to me.

Initially the mass was too big to operate on. She had to live with her breast while chemotherapy shrank the cancer to an operable size. During that time, she strode into new territory. Through meditation, she learned how to go into various parts of her body and talk with them. That is how she discovered her breasts' names, and how she learned that the breast with cancer was not a traitor, but was an embattled fighter who provided milk for the baby while trying and failing to keep the disease at bay. As Ellen came to know her breast, she came to love it and in this way worked through the emotions of losing it. Each step of the way, Ellen flooded herself with peace and strength and resolution.

When it came to appearance, however, there were problems. Consider bathing suits. For the same reasons turbans didn't cut it for her—they made her feel like a cancer patient—water wear designed specifically to accommodate mastectomies didn't go over too well either. She decided on a fashion line that included loose fitting jogging tops and bottoms from J. Crew.

She still had to tackle the dilemma of the vacancy created by the missing breast. Invoking falsies and wonderbras, I pointed out that this gave her something of a Hollywood opportunity to toy with her appearance out of necessity, which would reduce the peculiar shame attached to faking a figure. This point made no impression. The thought of a prosthesis continued to annoy her. How do you get it to stay in there? Will it float away in the water? Do you take it off at night and slap it on in the morning? Where do I buy one?

Needless to say, there is an Internet market for all this. Buyable breasts range from teardrops to pendulous and you can even get attachable nipples. By and large, post mastectomy products are covered by insurance.

At *Belle-Amie* (translated "beautiful friend"), you can have an impression of your chest taken before and/or after surgery to assure the right form. Their breast replicates the weight of a natural breast and is said to feel like real skin. The nipple, areola and breast itself are matched to your skin color. Their breast is completely removable and does not necessitate special clothing or pocket bras.

Company founder Janice M. Thielbar is a breast cancer survivor and a "medical artist". She

... she learned that the breast with cancer was not a traitor, but was an embattled fighter who provided milk for the baby while trying and failing to keep the disease at bay.

has studied fine art, makeup, special effects and prostheses at California State University, the Academy of Motion Picture Arts and Sciences, Tufts University and UCLA. Belle-Amie is headquartered in Los Angeles, California with a satellite office in Southfield, Michigan. Be forewarned: this level of expertise can be very expensive.

The breast forms at *ButterFly Image* are made of medical grade silicon and are also weighted.

The draw at *Ladies First, Inc.*, is their "Softee" Two top that has a "Roo" pocket for the post-mastectomy drainage tubes. Those pesky tubes gave Ellen some trouble. Ladies First has a variety of tops, some with pockets to hold the new breast. Their national sales representative, LuAnne Temple, is a breast cancer survivor.

Ready for this? *Lucy's Alternative Breast Implants* is sort of like the bargain basement for breast forms. Lucy's hits you with a challenge "to find the same models at a lower cost," and if you do, they'll undercut the price. Lucy's caters to the transgender crowd—pretty diverting if you chose to follow the links. In a way, it beats sentimentality. Lucy's has attachable "Nearly Me" silicone gel patches to help breast forms stay in place.

Shortly before the mastectomy, Ellen had a good-bye party for her breast which I missed because I was now trying quite hard to figure out what I was doing in New Mexico. (The party was a success—she told me she served pink coconut Hostess cupcakes because they resembled breast mounds and everyone loved them.)

After surgery, a portion of breast tissue was returned to her and she plans to have a ceremony—perhaps on her fortieth birthday—and a proper burial for it. While giving that part of herself back to the earth, Ellen will salute its effort and will grieve for the losses she and her breast suffered together.

Belle-Amie (http://www.belle-amie.com)
ButterFly Image (http://www.bfi-ia.com)
Ladies First, Inc (http://www.wvi.com/~ladies1)
Lucy's Alternative Breast Implants (http://www.lucys.net)

While giving that part of herself back to the earth, Ellen will salute its effort and will grieve for the losses she and her breast suffered together.

Learning to Look for Lymphedema

After her surgery, the drainage tubes poking into and out of her body disturbed Ellen. She didn't like to look at them. They hurt. They made sleeping difficult. Getting clothes to fit around them was a chore. No one seemed exactly sure when they could come out.

"The drains are draining," she wrote in her journal. She translated her dripping fluids into tears her body shed for what it had been through and for its missing breast.

Eventually, and pretty much on time, the tubes were taken out. Ellen's spirits lifted. The physical reminders of the disease and its consequences had proven a mighty challenge.

Still though, her arm hurt. One night, she told me, her strength failed as she was putting Stafford to bed. She barely managed a rousing toss-drop that completely canceled out the previous 20 minutes of lullabies.

Lymphedema was a scary threat. That's lymph-edema—"Ballooning Limb" Syndrome—an extremely serious, potential post-mastectomy complication that can, in rare cases, lead to amputation.

The *National Lymphedema Network* says: "Lymphedema is an accumulation of lymphatic fluid in the interstitial tissue that causes swelling, most often in the arm(s)..." It happens when the lymphatic system is impaired due to radiation or removal of lymph nodes.

Although lymphedema is a lifelong threat for breast cancer survivors and can strike any time—immediately after surgery or 30 years later—there is no standardized treatment for it in the United States, which can lead to trouble with insurance companies.

Lymphedema is preventable, not curable, and one of the best ways to prevent it is to learn about it. A great place to start is Bosom Buddies Breast Cancer Support, Inc (BBBCSI). The non-profit breast cancer and lymphedema support group serves women in Southwest Florida and if the world were a better place, there would be an organization like this in every community.

While not everyone can take advantage of all BBBCSI has to offer, everyone can read their excellent "Lymphedema Primer." Starting out at their Webpage will open up several lymphedema-related options including "Lymphedema Action Plan," "Lymphedema Prevention is Now," and "Use of Compression Pumps"—a discussion about a controversial treatment.

BBBCSI's material should be required reading. Their descriptions are more pointed than

She translated her dripping fluids into tears her body shed for what it had been through and for its missing breast.

most and their sharp angles provide insight you won't get from the other sites.

The non-profit National Lymphedema Network (NLN) was founded in 1988 by Saskia R.J. Thiadens to educate and help people with lymphedema, and to attempt to develop standardized quality treatment for lymphedema in the U.S. NLN lists support groups, treatment centers, diagnostic centers, and physicians who treat Lymphedema, alphabetically by state.

A British organization called *CancerBACUP* has put excerpts from their $7 booklet, "*Understanding Lymphedema*," on the Web. Chapters include "The Lymphatic system," "What is the treatment for lymphoedema?", "Compression garments," and "Limb positioning and movement" and others.

On their Website, the *National Alliance of Breast Cancer Organizations* (NABCO), established in 1986, offers information about cancers of all kinds and I found a concise article on lymphedema.

Healthworks, a clearinghouse for health and well-being information, products, and self-help education, has a two-pager—*Lymphedema FAQs*.

Days before Ellen went to Maine, she saw a psychic astrologer. Delirious with joy, she called me and announced: "I'm going to live! Betsy, I'm going to live!"

In Maine and on the advice of her 73-year-old neighbor, Ellen swam daily in the ocean. "If she can do it..." Ellen said.

Since Ellen had only one lymph node removed, she will probably not suffer from lymphedema. Others who are not so lucky will be restricted in many ways—shaving under the arm closest to their missing breast could be hazardous. Carrying a heavy shoulder bag won't be a good idea. Airplane cabin pressure could affect an impaired lymphatic system. Carelessly cradling a baby on that side will be ill-advised. Little things. It pays to remain vigilant.

The scar across her chest and the tattoos from radiation will be some of the only visible signs of her intensely trying experience. Ellen is lucky.

National Lymphedema Network (http://www.lymphnet.org)
CancerBACUP's "Understanding Lymphedema" page
    (http://www.cancerbacup.org.uk/info/lymphedema.htm)
National Alliance of Breast Cancer Organizations (http://www.nabco.org)
Healthworks' Lymphedema FAQs (http://www.pblsh.com/Healthworks/lymfaqs.html)

> *Delirious with joy, she called me and announced: "I'm going to live! Betsy, I'm going to live!"*

Considering Bone Marrow Transplants

The thought of a bone marrow transplant (BMT) leaves me cold with fear. To some doctors, the procedure smacks of unnecessary heroics. Others believe it saves lives. No one is wishy washy about bone marrow transplants (performed on people with blood cancers), or peripheral stem cell transplants (performed on people with other diseases, such as certain breast cancers).

Most women with ibc have to decide whether or not to have the procedure, yet all they know is that professional advice is divided and research to date has shown mixed results.

Sloan-Kettering thoroughly opposes the procedure. Ellen's local oncologist, however, says, "Bone marrow transplants save some people's lives. We just don't know who is going to benefit and you may be one of the lucky ones."

The only way to cut through the controversy is to learn about the procedure, its risk and consequences. I covered a lot of territory twice, but when "colony stimulating factors," "allogenic," "autologus," "purging" and other choice words made their way into my dinner table conversation, knowledge had put some of the fear to rest.

Although only a few online sites address bone marrow transplants specifically, they are thorough and give an excellent sense of the various hoops—and controversies—involved.

A good report to read first comes from *Emergency Care Research Institute* (ECRI), an independent, nonprofit watchdog organization concentrating on healthcare technology. In 1996—a long time ago in cancer research—ECRI staff wrote a *patient reference guide* to relevant published studies called "High-Dose Chemotherapy with Bone Marrow Transplant for Metastatic Breast Cancer." It's all online. Keep in mind it is only one side of the story.

Another book online, "*Bone Marrow Transplants*" offers a sobering glimpse of how changed someone's life will be after recovery. The *National Bone Marrow Transplant Link* has another resource guide. Worth reading in the name of leaving no stone unturned.

When I had the basic concepts and terms down, I read *Keren Stronach's guide to transplants*, "What To Expect And How To Get Through It." Keren knows. She has had two transplants.

BMT-TALK—an ongoing online discussion about bone marrow transplants—is another way to become familiar with BMT specifics. Another online chat is the *BMT Support Online*, where patients, caregivers and friends discuss their experiences.

> *... when "colony stimulating factors," "allogenic," "autologus," "purging" ... made their way into my dinner table conversation, knowledge had put some of the fear to rest.*

If the decision to get the transplant is made, the Blood & Marrow Transplant Newsletter offers a patient-to-survivor link. Complete the online questionnaire and in five days someone from the Newsletter will be in touch with you. If reading helps, imagine what real conversation can do.

One last thing—the National Bone Marrow Transplant Link is developing "A Companion Guide For Breast Cancer Patients."

For a list of hospitals performing transplants, check out the *Oncology Nursing Society*. They have a registration process that requires you list your mother's maiden name.

Unpleasantly vexed, Ellen struggled with her decision for months. She read. She talked with people who had chosen each option. No matter what she did, she still found that she didn't know how she felt. If she chose not to have it, was she just being overly confident? If she chose to have it, was she following that path out of fear? Up until then, her experience with cancer treatment and "cures" had not been the greatest.

She tried to set up a conference call between Dr. Hudis (against the procedure), Dr. Hendricks (sure that the procedure saved some lives, just didn't know whose) and a third doctor who had actually performed the procedure. The idea seemed a perfect way for Ellen to get the information she needed—an intellectual debate between the people she was entrusting her life to.

She ran the idea by Dr. Hudis, who said a telephone debate would degenerate into defensive posturing. But by then, Ellen had enough information. She decided not to have the procedure.

In lieu of a peripheral stem cell transplant, she will undergo a spiritual/emotional transplant, perhaps when she formally buries her breast tissue. She will spend time alone, in the desert or in a monastery. Then she will be baptized so that through ritual, those parts of her that must die will be washed away as her new body is being symbolically born into its new life.

ECRI Patient reference guide (http://www.hslc.org/emb/bc.txt)
Bone Marrow Transplants (http://www.bmtnews.org/bmt/bmt.book/toc.html)
The National Bone Marrow Transplant Link (http://comnet.org/nbmtlink)
Keren Stronach's guide to transplants (http://comnet.org/nbmtlink/sg.html)
BMT TALK (http://www.acor.org//listserv.html?to_do=interact&listname=BMT-TALK)
BMT Support Online (http://users.aol.com/kendrabmt/bmtonli.htm)
Oncology Nursing Society (http://www.ons.org)

Financing a Bone Marrow Transplant

Bone marrow transplants can cost more than $200,000—*not* including the costs of aftercare or medication. They can bankrupt families two ways—emotionally or financially (almost no insurance company covers transplant services without a long, drawn-out negotiation.)

Luckily there are a handful of organizations ready to help defray the costs of transplants or to help finance the cost of post-operative medications. If nothing else, some of these organizations will assign a patient advocate to your case—someone who knows how to deal with difficult insurance companies.

"The good news is that nine out of ten patients who persist will eventually be covered," writes Douglas Coleman in an article called, "No Need to Panic When Coverage Is Denied." I found the article at T*he Bone Marrow Foundation* and learned that some transplant centers have full-time transplant coordinators on staff dedicated to helping patients get coverage.

Another thing I didn't realize, but should have, is that some insurance companies will only cover the cost of a transplant if it is performed at the transplant center which gives them a discount.

To make life easier during the stress of transplant time, *The National Transplant Assistance Fund* (NTAF) offers an array of financial services. You can learn about NTAF from their Website, but to get financial aid, you need to call: 1-800-642-8399.

The *National Foundation for Transplants* (NFT), formerly Organ Transplant Fund, helps pay for post-transplant medications. Besides that, NFT will show you how to establish a fund-raising campaign (click the Reaching Out To Help box on their home page) if you need $10,000 or more for transplant-related costs. You'll get a patient advocate from their staff who will give you training, advice and consultation. If, for any reason, you can't reach them online you may want to call: 1-800-489-3863.

Most of these sites also explain how to donate an organ, marrow or money. I found a couple of sites that focus on facilitating body-part donations and have included them in case you are considering a donation. The National Marrow Donor Program makes it their business to get the right donated parts to the right patient. I cut through the bells and whistles on their home page by clicking on the NMDP logo in the upper left-hand corner of the page, right at the top of

> *If nothing else, some of these organizations will assign a patient advocate to your case—someone who knows how to deal with difficult insurance companies.*

the curvy graphic. That got me to a no-frills contents page and I just moved through each "chapter" until I'd learned enough.

If you are a physician, *Bone Marrow Donors Worldwide* is a clearinghouse that links physicians scouting for their patients-in-need with actual donors. It's a well-designed site—clear and easy to use. Participating is made extremely easy.

Good luck.

The Bone Marrow Foundation (http://www.bonemarrow.org/panic.html)
The National Transplant Assistance Fund (http://www.transplantfund.org/answer4.html)
The National Foundation for Transplants (http://www.transplants.org)
The National Marrow Donor Program (http://www.marrow.org/2ndpage.html)
Bone Marrow Donors Worldwide (http://www.bmdw.org)

... Bone Marrow Donors Worldwide is a clearinghouse that links physicians scouting for their patients-in-need with actual donors.

Accepting the Prospect of Death

Another figure from childhood who played a role in Ellen's run with cancer was a man named Clay Kanzler. When we were all children, Clay was two or three years ahead of Ellen in school. He was a presence. By the time Ellen got sick, Clay's journey had forged him into a man of God and a successful artist living in Vermont.

He came to see Ellen several times and in his own words, "blasted her." He did this to many people fighting illness and brought the light and power of God into their living rooms.

"I'm looking for nothing less than a miracle," he told me one night after he'd been to Ellen's.

During the early days of Ellen's illness, Clay was staying at my father's house in Michigan, going out in the daytime and praying with and for Annie Peabody. Annie was in her early thirties. She had colon cancer. Annie died a month or so later. No one rushed to tell Ellen.

Not long enough after that, 27-year-old Sabra Dalby, also from our hometown, died of melanoma. Ellen had been Sabra's day-camp counselor years before. They did not see each other for almost 20 years, until they crossed paths at Sloan-Kettering in May. Ellen was there for her mastectomy. Sabra was there for what turned out to be one of her final visits. She died two weeks later on the plane ride home.

When Sabra died, Ellen called me. By this time I had migrated to Montana. The enormity of these two deaths had rocked Ellen's world. As Ellen's camper, Sabra once sank like a stone (Ellen's words) in the pool at the city park, almost drowning. Ellen saved her. Now Sabra was dead. From cancer.

Ellen struggled with what it all meant. Many people live through it, I told her—not Sabra... not Annie. There was no denying these deaths haunted Ellen, and everyone else, deeply. But especially Ellen. She knew, she said, that as time went on, she would have to find a way to handle other peoples' cancer deaths. And she will, with time and experience.

In the beginning, Ellen had to come to terms with accepting the prospect of death and fighting tooth and nail to keep her life. The loss of even younger women whom she knew changed the challenge. Ellen has to find a way to keep their deaths, and those that will follow, from diminishing her sense of purpose and her sense of belonging.

This is such a private issue—making peace with death—there are no adequate Websites, but

... Ellen had to come to terms with accepting the prospect of death and fighting tooth and nail to keep her life.

National Public Radio's site "*The End of Life: Exploring Death in America*" comes close. Articles like "*Learning to Live Again: AIDS patient embraces recovery after making peace with death*," in the Dallas Morning News, can also be powerful.

    After the mastectomy, the Graysons went to Maine where the prospect of death and dying loomed less large for Ellen.

"It was so in my face in D.C. Here, it doesn't feel as urgent," she said. "Stafford's hair is turning blonde in the sun." Ellen is engaged in the world around her.

"It's nice to be playing a little right now," she continued. "But the whole death issue is something I need to look at closely without fear. Hang on a minute—oh shoot, I just checked the clock. I've got to get Stafford into her swimming diapers. We're late for the beach!"

In the morning, Ellen nestles Stafford into her stroller and they walk to the Giant Steps, a rock formation of natural risers that lead to a magnificent crest overlooking the crashing sea. "I stand there with Stafford and I pray to the sea and to everyone who is helping me. Stafford loves it there," Ellen told me later, "and I feel cleansed."

National Public Radio
    "The End of Life: Exploring Death in America" (http://www.npr.org/programs/death)
Dallas Morning News
    "Learning to Live Again: AIDS patient embraces recovery after making peace with death" (http://www.aegis.com/news/dmn/1999/DN990101.html)

"... Stafford loves it there," Ellen told me later, "and I feel cleansed."

Preparing for Menopause

"So what's your head like? Is there hair?" I ask from Montana.

"I totally have hair. I guess you'd have to call it boy hair at this point," Ellen says.

"Are you sleeping? How are the hot flashes?" I ask.

"Better. I've gotten a little more used to them," she says.

Ellen has menopause.

She wanted children very, very much. In an ideal world, she would have lots of them. Not being fertile shattered her. Both she and her two sisters resorted to infertility treatments to induce pregnancy, although Pam, the youngest, eventually got pregnant without such treatments.

Ellen and Roger embarked on a months-long journey of injections and doctor's appointments and egg harvests and hormonal roller coasters and daunting questions and finally, in a test tube, they got what would become Stafford. Stafford was late and almost died during her birth. The cord was wrapped around her neck and she was not properly attached to the placenta. Ellen had an emergency C-section.

Less than a year later, Ellen started going through menopause—a side effect of her chemotherapy. A couple of weeks after she realized this was going to happen, her little sister announced her second pregnancy. On the phone with Pam, Ellen cried with joy and rage.

For months, the hot flashes have thoroughly disrupted her sleep. Adequate sleep helps keep her strong. She's also gained some weight—a major victory for someone getting chemotherapy—but she doesn't want to lose her new and trim figure. Vaginal dryness is a problem. Sexuality simply takes a back seat when all these other things are happening.

When Ellen talks about this angle, there is an apologetic note in her voice towards Roger. Neither of them could have foreseen the length of time she was going to be out of commission—from pregnancy through breast cancer, she says. It will be a relief for them both, she explains, when she is able to stop focusing so intensely on her own self.

Early menopause is a common side effect of chemotherapy for young women with breast cancer. It can be a shock, so prepare yourself to live through it. You can't reverse it yourself, but on occasion, in breast cancer patients, menopause does reverse itself.

Reading about menopause is a lot like reading the back of tampon boxes before reaching

> *Reading about menopause is a lot like reading the back of tampon boxes before reaching puberty.*

puberty. The tone of most written material gives the impression of something strange and mysterious and not altogether pleasant.

Discussions of induced menopause, which Ellen has, are something of a rarity, but *The North American Menopause Society* has a couple of paragraphs on it at their Website.

For a basic rundown on what menopause is and what to expect, go to Chapter 28 of the *Physician's Desk Reference Family Guide to Women's Health*. It's all about menopause and has a most unsettling section called, "Changes to Expect," things like sagginess and brittle bones.

Another good place to look is at the *Mayo Clinic's Health Oasis Website for Women's Health*. When I was last there, I found 17 articles addressing different aspects of menopause, from sexuality to weight gain.

"*What Can I Do About Hot Flashes And Night Sweats*," an article by Madelon Hope, talks about herbal alternatives to hormone replacement therapy, which might be useful for women with induced menopause. Hope mentions several remedies.

The *Doctor's Guide Menopause Information and Resources* Webpage, sponsored by P\S\L Consulting Group Inc., has loads of stuff—medical articles, news flashes, plus links to discussion groups and related sites. P\S\L is sponsored by the likes of Eli Lilly, Glaxo-Wellcome and Bristol-Myers Squibb Company. Their menopause page is well stocked.

Once in the middle of this whole episode, I was overcome not only by the number of issues Ellen had to plow through, but also their emotional difficulty. Tears welled in my eyes and I said, "I'm so sorry you have to go through all this."

Ellen looked at me without a touch of sentiment and said, "Why? It is my path."

The North American Menopause Society (http://www.menopause.org/pfaq.htm)
Physician's Desk Reference Family Guide to Women's Health
  (http://www.healthsquare.com/pdrfg/wh/chapters/wh1ch28.htm)
Mayo Clinic's Health Oasis Website for Women's Health
  (http://www.mayohealth.org/mayo/common/htm/womenpg2.htm)
Madelon Hope's article, "What Can I Do About Hot Flashes And Night Sweats"
  (http://world.std.com/~susan207/flash.html)
P\S\L Consulting Group Inc.'s Doctor's Guide—Menopause Information and Resources
  (http://www.pslgroup.com/MENOPAUSE.HTM)

Tears welled in my eyes and I said, "I'm so sorry you have to go through all this."

Ellen looked at me without a touch of sentiment and said, "Why? It is my path."

Uncovering Male Breast Cancer

Since Ellen's cancer was diagnosed, she has talked with other women who have, or have had, breast cancer. So have I. Neither of us have ever talked to a man who has breast cancer, but male breast cancer accounts for one out of every 100 breast cancer cases in the United States.

Men are usually older when their cancer is diagnosed. They tend to discover the painless lump in their breast themselves, not with the help of a mammogram. Diagnosis is often delayed. Since the notion of having breast cancer can strike at the heart of masculinity, men tend not to see a doctor immediately. Black men seem more at risk than white men. In general, men respond well to hormone therapy. They sometimes have reconstructive surgery.

A handful of sites address male breast cancer, but without the same passion and informational bounty that women have fought to enjoy. In fact, I had to visit Alexandra Andrews's site, cancerlinks.org, to find any information at all.

Two sites I saw outdid all the others: a write-up by Dr. Carol Scott-Conner of the *University of Iowa Hospitals and Clinics* Department of Surgery; and the *Komen Foundation* male breast cancer page.

The former has a thorough fact sheet discussing causes, incidence, treatment, and answers all the most obvious initial questions. It also has two important links to further discussions, one for gynecomastia (the term for the male breast becoming overdeveloped), which is sometimes misdiagnosed as breast cancer; and one for reconstructive surgery. The article is well footnoted, so the source material can be easily obtained.

The Komen Foundation is a service of the Susan G. Komen Breast Cancer Foundation—the Race for the Cure people. The male breast cancer page, which employs bullets, is designed to convey critical information succinctly—What are the signs? What are the risk factors? Is the survival rate better for men?—and so on. If you can't access the page using the first address listed, try the second and click on "Male breast cancer" in the right hand column.

Male Breast Cancer, Information Center, developed in 1995, is dedicated to those who have died and to those currently fighting male breast cancer. This is the only Website devoted entirely to male breast cancer that I found and for that reason it is a stand-out. Almost everything you'd want to know at first blush is gathered under the "About" heading. "Frequently Asked Questions" is sparse. "Medical References" has been growing recently; that is where you may submit

... male breast cancer accounts for one out of every 100 breast cancer cases in the United States.

a form to join a male breast cancer online support group. In addition, this site offers a list of good links that mainly take you to other sites addressing cancer-in-general or female breast cancer.

Y-ME National Breast Cancer Organization, created in 1978 by two women with breast cancer to provide information to anyone impacted by breast cancer, has a male breast cancer page. The information is not too abundant and is not startlingly different from what you can find elsewhere, but it never hurts to look.

Another place to look is the *Imperial Cancer Research Fund's* page. The Imperial Cancer Research Fund (ICRF), a registered charity in the United Kingdom, is "dedicated to saving lives through research into the causes, prevention, treatment and cure of cancer." Right off the bat, you find out that in the UK, men afflicted with breast cancer have high survival rates, which is comforting to read. In the UK, the ICRF is responsible for more than one-third of all cancer research, which is also comforting to read.

Last but not least is the *Breast Cancer Information Services* (BCIS) male breast cancer page. BCIS is a "joint project of the Pittsburgh Breast Care Test Coalition, an umbrella organization of health care providers, women's groups and individuals dedicated to the eradication of breast cancer as a life-threatening disease." You may find information here you have not seen elsewhere.

The shame of the situation is that so very many women had to suffer breast cancer before good research was undertaken and subsequently good information became available. With luck, men will benefit equally from the lessons learned in their sisters' struggle.

> Male breast cancer, Department of Surgery, The University of Iowa Hospitals and Clinics
> (http://www.surgery.uiowa.edu/surgery/oncology/malebreastcancer.html)
> The Komen Foundation
> (http://www.breastcancerinfo.com/bhealth/html/male_breast_cancer.asp)
> Male Breast Cancer, Information Center (http://interact.withus.com/interact/mbc)
> Y-ME National Breast Cancer Organization (http://www.y-me.org/malebc2.html)
> Imperial Cancer Research Fund (http://www.lif.icnet.uk/research/factsheet/malebreast.html)
> Breast Cancer Information Services (http://trfn.clpgh.org/bcis/GeneralInfo/male.html)

With luck, men will benefit equally from the lessons learned in their sisters' struggle.

Investigating Environmental Estrogens

Ellen and I both had heard there was a connection between estrogen and breast cancer. I set out to learn more.

If you're involved with breast cancer, most likely you've also heard words like "endocrine disrupters" or "environmental estrogens." Some believe there is a link between breast cancer and other cancers of the reproductive organs and hormones like estrogen, but pinning down the exact relationship is tricky.

In fact, there is currently a massive debate about the very existence of a relationship. The sides are polarized: either environmental estrogens don't disrupt the endocrine system and have nothing to do with reproductive (breast) cancers, or they have everything to do with such cancers.

The debate and polarization are worth noting because although there are places to go to learn about this subject, sources tend to take one side or the other. I am going to lead you to sites where the information suggests that there is often a relationship between environmental estrogens and breast cancer. I believe the truth lies on that side of the debate.

To be moderately fair, however, there is a site that provides a readable, balanced explanation of environmental estrogens and endocrine disrupters. A joint effort of the Center for Bioenvironmental Research of Tulane and Xavier Universities (CBR), in New Orleans, Louisiana, it is packed with information regarding environmental estrogen and spin-off subjects, like steroid hormones and phytoestrogens and synthetic chemicals.

For a short description about what the Center is up to as far as environmental estrogens are concerned, go to their *Environmental Endocrinology* Webpage. One of their primary concerns, as you will read, is women's health.

To see a good rundown on the whole issue of environmental estrogens, which the Center defines as "Substances that act like estrogen hormones in living organisms...", go to their Environmental Estrogens and Other Hormones page. The options on the left serve as chapter heads that take you to two- or three-page briefs, each of which has links to deeper definitions woven into longer articles.

If you have any doubts that environmental estrogens are and have been a subject of concern for some time, see the Center's *Milestone* Webpage, where there is a timeline following environmental hormone research from 1923 to 1998.

Another reliable place, with more of an activist bent, for reading about environmental estrogens and *endocrine disrupters* is The World Wildlife Fund (WWF).

At their site I learned "Some endocrine disrupting chemicals are persistent in the environment and bioaccumulate; they accumulate in the fatty tissue of organisms and increase in concentration as they move up through the food Web. Because of their persistence and mobility, they accumulate in and harm species far from their original source." This site is opinionated, but since breasts contain a lot of fatty tissue I find the association compelling. Follow the prompts and you will get a short report on the subject.

Lastly, the nonprofit Institute for Agriculture and Trade Policy (IATP) has an *Endocrine Disrupter Resources* of many types. It is strangely organized, but you will find a list by clicking Related sites, then selecting Endocrine Disrupter Information from the pull down menu.

The same pull down menu allows you to visit lists of links to environmental, scientific, healthcare industry and trade organizations, environmental justice groups, universities, online publications and more.

One of the questions in Ellen's case is: Did the fertility drugs—which boost estrogen levels—that she took contribute to the growth of her breast cancer?

It's a hard question, not because answering it is tricky or even possible—but because sometimes drifting off to sleep it's hard not to wonder.

On Roger's birthday I called Maine to wish him a happy one. Stafford, he reported, walked into the ocean up to her chest that day. Then, he said, Ellen took Stafford's hands in hers and swooped her around in great big circles.

CBR Environmental Endocrinology (http://www.tmc.tulane.edu/cbr/research/endocrinology.html)
CBR Environmental Estrogens and Other Hormones
    (http://www.tmc.tulane.edu/ECME/eehome/basics/estrogen)
CBR Milestone page (http://www.tmc.tulane.edu/ECME/eehome/sources/milestones)
WWF Endocrine Disrupters page (http://worldwildlife.org/toxics/progareas/ed/index.htm)
IATP Endocrine Disrupter Resource Center (http://www.sustain.org/hcwh/main.htm)

"Some endocrine disrupting chemicals ... bioaccumulate ... in the fatty tissue of organisms ... increase in concentration as they move up through the food Web ... and harm species far from their original source."

Pondering Environmental Carcinogens

After Ellen and I realized the kind of retreat we had envisioned creating already existed in Commonweal, our thoughts about how to give back diverged. With what energy she had to spare, Ellen focused primarily on getting herself better. I started wondering why so many people had cancer.

I discovered that a growing number of respected and credentialed scientists and researchers contend that certain toxic chemicals mimic estrogens in our bodies and that high estrogen levels often lead to breast (and other) cancer.

Serendipitously or not, books and articles about carcinogenic environmental toxins began falling into my hands. Some of the most credible and chilling information I saw specifically about breast cancer came from World Resources Institute (WRI), a Washington, D.C. based organization created in 1982 to encourage both a healthy environment and strong economy.

In an article written by Dr. Devra Lee Davis, Deborah Axelrod, Michael P. Osborne and Nitin T. Telang (originally published in Science and Medicine,) I read: "Fewer than 10% of breast cancers develop because of inherited genetic defects, and known risk factors do not explain most sporadic cases. Excepting radiation.... Cumulative exposure to estrogen underlies most of the known risk factors for breast cancer..." To read the whole article, go to the WRI posting of *"Environmental Influences on Breast Cancer Risks."*

Another WRI site, the *Health and Environment Webpage*, has a variety of relevant topics such as "Environmental Links to Breast Cancer and Other Reproductive Health Problems," and "Missing Baby Boys—Reduced Ratio of Male to Female Births in Several Industrial Countries: A Sentinel Health Indicator," and "Stresses on Ecosystem Health: Chemical Pollution."

While these titles may sound like the same old ranting we've been hearing from environmentalists since the late sixties, the science and the documented findings will not—largely because we have now had 30 years of results.

If any of this entices you, a third WRI site, their *Business and Environment Resources Worldwide Webpage*, offers a bountiful array of interesting environmental links where you can learn about everything from corporate pollution emissions, to which specific toxic contaminants are floating around in your municipal tap water.

I started wondering why so many people had cancer.

Not surprisingly, Commonweal also has a handful of riveting, well written and well documented sites relating to environmental influences and topics. If you go to their main page and scroll down, you will see them. Health Care without Harm, a Commonweal campaign, is "an inspiring grass-roots-based, national campaign to end dioxin and mercury pollution from medical waste incineration.... Both dioxin and mercury are potent developmental and reproductive toxins. Dioxin is also a carcinogen: it causes cancer."

There is also news about "POPS: The United Nations Environment Program Treaty Process on Persistent Organic Pollutants." It's burdensomely technical, but if you scan it, you'll get the idea that something out there may be a little out of whack.

All these sites might be of interest if you even suspect that environmental contaminants play a role in the causation of cancer. If you happen to agree with this premise already and want to learn more about how to protect your own self, *Mothers & Others*, a national nonprofit education organization, can steer you away from problematic products on the market to safer alternatives. Even if you don't like the tone, the facts are useful. Actress Meryl Streep is a co-founder.

In the midst of looking at all these sites, I read a book called "Living Downstream," by Sandra Steingraber, a scientist and survivor of a bladder cancer. Her incredible book, complete with detailed source notes, picks up where Rachel Carson's "Silent Spring" left off, making the persuasive argument that environmental carcinogens clearly play a role in many of the cancers we see around us.

Ellen's susceptibility to cancer was probably heightened by the radiation she received for Hodgkin's, but what about other people's cancers? Do environmental toxins influence the development and growth of cancer?

If that is even a possibility, is that okay?

WRI's "Environmental Influences on Breast Cancer Risks" (http://www.wri.org/health/med-e-br.html)
WRI's Health and Environment Webpage (http://www.wri.org/health)
WRI's Business and Environment Resources Worldwide Webpage (http://www.wri.org/meb/links.html)
Mothers & Others (http://www.mothers.org)

Ellen's susceptibility to cancer was probably heightened by the radiation she received for Hodgkin's, but what about other people's cancers?

Taking Action for a Change

Activism is not for everyone. I don't think it's for Ellen.

Right now she needs to think almost exclusively about herself. Naturally she's also thinking about her family, Stafford and Roger, but she invests the majority of whatever energy and time she has straight back into herself. She writes, meditates, prays, walks, paints . . . these tasks amount to her homework. In addition to her chemo, finished in September, Ellen had six weeks of radiation and endured the resulting low energy. Then there's the food: nothing is instant and nothing is fast. Preparation to clean up can take hours, three times a day. Priscilla helps with dinner, but that leaves two other meals.

Even when she's finished with treatment, Ellen is probably not going to put her extra time into activism. It's not where her heart lies. Some people, however, do want to politicize their experience with cancer. Sometimes it's a sister or daughter or friend who concludes that taking action is the best way to respond to cancer.

If this is your path, you should know that there are organizations that are dedicated to advocacy. For the most part, their major goals involve education and then eradication of breast cancer one way or the other. That may sound lofty, but when you consider that since the early sixties, a woman's chance of getting breast cancer has moved from one in twenty, to one in eight, you get the feeling that perhaps the pattern can be reversed. Whether you give time or money, advocacy has its place.

Established in 1990 by a handful of breast cancer survivors, the California-based *Breast Cancer Action* is a good place to bone up on what's going on out there. Breast Cancer Action "carries the voices of people affected by breast cancer to inspire and compel the changes necessary to end the breast cancer epidemic." You can read pointed articles about hot button issues, such as the direct marketing of certain cancer-related drugs like tamoxifen and raloxifene. Together with a number of other advocacy groups, Breast Cancer Action is planning to tackle that very issue and they could use help.

Also in California, *The Breast Cancer Fund* intends to "change the way people think about breast cancer – from personal tragedy to public health crisis. . ." They have an excellent site. Stressing the role environmental contaminants play in the existence of cancer, The Breast Cancer Fund (TBCF) site has good powerful articles: "Understanding the Language of Cancer and

... since the early sixties, a woman's chance of getting breast cancer has moved from one in twenty, to one in eight ...

Environmental Connections," "Searching for Environmental Causes of Breast Cancer," "Unacceptable Risk: PVC Plastic in Medical Products," "Possible Breast Carcinogen Found In Human Milk," and more.

Founded in 1992 by breast cancer survivor Andrea Martin, TBCF participates in the *Lilith Fair* and also created a national campaign called, "Climb Against The Odds." By ascending some of the world's most challenging mountains, breast cancer survivors raise "hope, awareness and funding. . ." Getting involved with TBCF is as easy as clicking the box that says, "A Call To Action."

The Women's Environment and Development Organization (WEDO) is "an international advocacy network actively working to transform society to achieve a healthy and peaceful planet. . ." To those ends, WEDO has an Action Plan for Cancer Prevention Campaign working on many levels to publicize the rampant nature of breast cancer and to arrest it. If you browse their site, you will find ways to get involved.

Has everyone heard of the National *Race for the Cure* by now? Founded by the Susan G. Komen Breast Cancer Foundation, it's the biggest five kilometer walk/run in the U.S. and it pulls down a great deal of money that goes into the fight against breast cancer. The Race began with 7,000 participants back in 1990 and by 1999, a total of 66,000 people went for it. If you want to get involved you can run, you can walk and you can volunteer your services.

If participating in the crusade against breast cancer is what you want to do, you'll find many more options than have been mentioned here. Local organizations have sprung up everywhere and they need hands and help, too.

In Maine, Ellen is in touch with a woman who had breast cancer long ago. The woman, Sally Walbridge, has written a book about breast cancer resources in and for her local community. Sally is involved in other ways as well.

But Ellen doesn't want to do that. She just wants to put it all behind her and will be happy when this experience is a distant memory.

    Breast Cancer Action (http://www.bcaction.org)
    The Breast Cancer Fund (http://www.breastcancerfund.org)
    Lilith Fair (http://www.lilithfair.com)
    The Women's Environment and Development Organization (http://www.wedo.org)
    The Susan G. Komen Breast Cancer Foundation National Race for the Cure
        (http://www.natl-race-for-the-cure.org)

Local organizations have sprung up everywhere and they need hands and help, too.

Hoodwinked!

One day before chemo, Ellen and I were in my kitchen happily testing fresh hummus on non-wheat crackers. When the time came to leave, we walked to her car, and both saw it at the same moment: another parking ticket. It seemed so unfair. Just when you think you have life's major stresses under control, fate steps in and you get another reality check.

So it was on another day as we hurried home after a chemo session, whizzing along a windy Washington road heading towards Key Bridge. Ellen, in the driver's seat, was talking about what she had been learning from her spiritual advisor when suddenly she got paler than I thought possible.

"Oh no," she whispered, as the dreaded flashing blue lights of a police car appeared in the rear view mirror. "It's a cop."

She started pulling over. A ticket was going to be expensive—exactly what she and Roger didn't need. If she hadn't morphed into a high-maintenance gal, it wouldn't have mattered. A pit lodged in our mutual stomach and we looked at each other and said, "What do we do now?" As Ellen edged towards the curb and started rolling down her window, I stared at my lap hoping an idea would form somewhere near my kneecap.

"Quick—get the scarf off your head," I said.

She looked at me incredulously. "What?"

"Take it off. You've got cancer. You just had chemotherapy. You're distracted."

Ellen whipped off the scarf just in time to present her resplendently bald head to the policeman—and played the sympathy card full-tilt, except it was all real.

"Officer, I've recently been diagnosed with inflammatory breast cancer. I am driving home from getting chemotherapy. I have to relieve the 70-year-old babysitter of my nine-month-old daughter. And I'm late. Please—I'm sorry. It won't happen again."

He gaped, sweetly, and wished her luck.

I asked her later how she interpreted what had happened.

"I thought, 'Goodie!'" she laughed.

"We sure hoodwinked him! He really thought one of us was sick!"

> *Ellen whipped off the scarf just in time to present her resplendently bald head to the policeman—and played the sympathy card full-tilt ...*

VISIT US ONLINE @ FIRSTAIDYOURSELF.ORG

Glossary

abstracts – summaries of full medical or research reports.

accrual – the number of patients to be treated in a specific clinical trial. "Projected accrual 9" means that nine patients will be treated in a specific trial. "Accrual completed" means that those conducting a clinical trial have chosen the patients they will treat and no new patients are likely to be considered for treatment in that trial.

acupuncture – A medical therapy that originated in China more than 3000 years ago. It involves inserting needles into the skin at precise points and is commonly used in the West to control pain and the symptoms of illness. The National Institutes of Health deems it an effective treatment for nausea resulting from pregnancy, surgery, chemotherapy and dental procedures.

acupuncturist – one who administers acupuncture. Most states require acupuncturists to be licensed. A few allow only medical doctors and doctors of osteopathy to practice acupuncture. For more information, visit Acupuncture.com at http://www.acupuncture.com.

adjuvant – serving to aid or contribute; one that helps or facilitates, especially something that enhances the effectiveness of medical treatment. "Adjuvant" chemotherapy uses additional drugs for patients with cancers that are believed to have spread beyond their original site.

adriamycin (doxorubicin) – An anthracycline antibiotic used in chemotherapy to disrupt the growth of cancer cells, which are then destroyed.

biofeedback – a process in which a person consciously regulates bodily functions such as blood pressure, heart rate, muscle tension and temperature. The mind's control of these physical functions is demonstrated with monitoring instruments so the person may learn how to influence responses commonly considered to be involuntary.

biopsy – the removal and examination of sample tissue, cells or fluids from the living body to see whether cancer cells are present.

bone marrow transplants – a treatment in which some of a patient's or donor's bone marrow is removed from the patient (autologous) or donor (allogenic), cleaned, treated and stored. Once the marrow has been withdrawn, the patient receives very high doses of chemotherapy to destroy as many cancer cells as possible. These high doses also destroy the remaining bone marrow, which the body relies upon to fight infection. After the chemotherapy has been administered, the stored marrow is returned to the patient by a transfusion or transplant.

cancer – a malignant tumor characterized by potentially unlimited growth with local expansion by invasion and systemic by metastasis; an enlarged tumor-like growth; a disease marked by such growth.

carcinogens – substances or agents producing or inciting cancer.

chemosensitivity testing – also known as "cell culture resistance testing." A patient's cancer cells are tested in a laboratory with various chemotherapeutic agents to see which drugs are most effective.

chemotherapy – the use of chemical agents in the treatment or control of disease (cancer).

clinical trials – research studies used to test new drugs or treatments. New treatments are studied in the lab before they are used on people. If a treatment proves viable in the lab, it is then tested on people. These human studies are called clinical trials.

Coenzyme Q 10 – a substance widely known as an electron carrier in the mitochondrial respiratory chain. Considered to be a powerful antioxidant, it is found in its highest concentrations in the heart and liver. The body synthesizes this substance.

complementary – mutually supplying each other's lack; serving to fill out or complete. "Complementary" therapies are those that are used along with conventional medical treatments to treat an illness or symptom; examples include meditation, yoga and acupuncture.

complementary and alternative treatments – "Complementary" refers to supportive methods used in conjunction with conventional treatments and intended to complement those treatments. Depending upon who is speaking, "alternative" can mean the same thing, or it can refer to treatments that have not been scientifically tested and are therefore considered largely unworthy or unsafe.

cooperatives – a program of combined studies at different institutions.

cultivated tumor cells – a process for growing human tumor-derived cells in a culture. These cells react to various chemotherapy drugs so the drugs' effectiveness may be measured.

cure – to restore to health, soundness or normality; to bring about recovery; heal.

cybercafe – a café offering the use of computers for a fee.

diagnosis – a statement or conclusion concerning the nature or cause of some phenomenon.

dioxin – a chemical by-product that is the result of heating combinations of chlorine and organic compounds; dioxin is produced, for example, when pulp paper is bleached, when materials containing chlorine compounds are incinerated and during the production of some pesticides.

dose-dense protocol – rapidly sequenced high-dose chemotherapy treatments.

dried blackberry – sometimes used as a remedy for diarrhea.

endocrine disrupters – chemicals that can disrupt normal cellular development by interfering with hormones and/or hormonal activity; endocrine disruption has been implicated as a possible

essiac tea – a mixture of herbs containing Burdock root, Turkish rhubarb, sheep sorrel and slipper elm tree bark. A nurse in Canada, Rene Caisse, named the tea after herself—it is her name spelled backwards.

estrogen – a female sex hormone primarily made by the ovaries and also by the adrenal cortex to some degree; women's estrogen levels fluctuate; this hormone is responsible for the development of secondary sex characteristics, such as breasts, and it regulates menstruation cycles; estrogen may promote the growth of cancer cells in breast cancer.

fertility drugs – drugs used to stimulate the potential for conception. In males, thyroid and, on occasion, pituitary hormones are frequently used. In females, gonadotropic hormones and, on occasion, clomiphene citrate are used.

grading – a system that reflects a cancer's degree of abnormality; pathologists "grade" cancer tissues by examining a biopsy.

gynecomastia – from the Greek words that mean "women-like breasts." An estimated 40 – 60% of men are affected and may be affected in one or both breasts. Breast reconstruction can ease the situation.

high-dose chemotherapy – a chemotherapy treatment plan using unusually high levels of drugs intended to destroy as many cancer cells as possible. High-dose chemotherapy also kills healthy blood cells and so is usually given in conjunction with a bone marrow transplant.

Hodgkin's disease – a type of cancer that starts in the lymphatic tissue.

hormone replacement therapy – the introduction of estrogen and progesterone from an external source after a woman's body has ceased to produce either hormone naturally or from induced menopause.

ibc – see "inflammatory breast cancer".

Iceland moss (Cetraria islandica) – a lichen used by some to treat various ailments such as coughs, fevers and scurvy.

immunology-based drugs – drugs that stimulate the body's ability to resist infection and disease.

in vitro fertilization (ivf) – is a process in which a woman's egg production is stimulated by a series of hormone injections or oral medications; at the best time for fertilization, eggs are harvested from the woman's ovary; in a lab, these eggs are mixed with sperm treated to maximize their fertilization capacities; if a fertilized egg results, it is transferred to the woman's uterus.

inflammatory breast cancer (ibc) – an infrequent form of breast cancer; symptoms usually include:
- The sudden appearance of a large lump in the breast
- Itching or pain in the breast
- A nipple which is flattened or inverted, possibly with a discharge
- Swollen lymph nodes under the arm or above the collarbone
- Reddish, dimpled-appearing skin resembling an orange skin
- A swollen warm breast.

inflammatory ductal carcinoma – an invasive cancer (meaning it has spread beyond its origins) that starts in the breast ducts, the route through which milk travels.

infusion – the act of introducing a solution into a vein.

Internet – information resources electronically accessible from remote locations.

kashi – a blend of sesame and seven whole grains, developed by Philip and Gayle Tauber in 1984. The name "Kashi" is a combination of "kashruth" or kosher, and "Kushi," the last name of the founders of a way of eating that involves whole foods, called Macrobiotics.

kosher – sanctioned by Jewish law; ritually fit for use.

lactation – to secrete milk.

latissimus – a primary back muscle.

leukemia – an acute or chronic disease of unknown cause in man and other warm-blooded animals characterized by an abnormal increase in the number of leukocytes in the tissues and often in the blood.

leukocytes – any of the white or colorless nucleated cells that occur in the blood.

lymphedema – a post-radiation or post-mastectomy complication that can involve swelling in the arm resulting from excess lymph fluid that builds up after lymph nodes and blood vessels have been either treated or removed.

mass – a quantity or aggregate of matter usually of considerable size.

mastectomy – excision or amputation of the breast.

mastitis – inflammation of the breast usually caused by infection.

meditation – the act of engaging in contemplation or reflection; a mind-body process which can produce physiological benefits.

melanoma – a usually malignant tumor containing dark pigment.

menopause – the period of natural cessation of menstruation occurring usually between the ages of 45 and 50.

nausea – a stomach distress with loathing for food and an urge to vomit.

neutropenia – a blood disorder involving low white blood cell counts which some people are born with, but which can also result from chemotherapy; neutropenia may lead to dangerous infections and in some cases may be life-threatening.

nutrition – the act or process of nourishing or being nourished; the sum of the processes by which an animal or plant takes in and utilizes food substances.

oncologist – a doctor with a special training in the diagnosis and treatment of cancer.

online discussion groups – discussions held electronically via the Internet between a variety of people with similar interests; information and ideas are disseminated over the Internet via online discussion groups.

organic – in popular usage, "organic" refers to food grown and produced without the use of synthetic chemicals, including manufactured antibiotics, pesticides, hormones; when the word "organic" is used in a discussion involving chemistry, however, it means a chemical that has carbon in it (see dioxin); organic chemicals are often synthetic.

peripheral stem cell transplant – procedure in which stem cells are collected from a patients bloodstream, stored and re-infused after the patient has been treated with high doses of chemotherapy to restore bone marrow function.

petri dish – a small shallow dish of thin glass with a loose cover used especially for cultures in bacteriology.

phytoestrogens – estrogens produced by plants.

protocol – a code of precedence or procedure; a cancer treatment plan, in detail, which includes the schedule and dose of drugs to be used.

pvc plastic – vinyl, or polyvinylchloride. Some products made of PVC include credit cards, some lawn furniture, some food-packaging materials. The vinyl chloride from which it is manufactured is a known human carcinogen. PVC plastic relies on a plasticizers called phthalates, which have been implicated in the disruption of the endocrine system.

radiation – the process of treating cancer by emitting radiant energy in the form of waves or particles, in this case to destroy cancer cells; treatment of this nature may be used to reduce the size of a tumor or to destroy it altogether.

recurrence – to occur again after an interval; cancer that has returned after treatment is said to have recurred; it may recur at the same site at which it was originally found or at a distant site.

remission – the act or process of giving relief from suffering; a period during which the signs and symptoms of cancer either fully or partially vanish. During remission, the disease is said to "be under control."

search – in this case, to instigate an electronic investigation of material concealed on the Internet, at a Website or within a document on a Website.

secondary breast cancer – a breast cancer that is the result of a spreading of the original tumor.

specialist – one who devotes himself to a special occupation or branch of learning.

staging – a process that determines if and how far the cancer has spread. There is more than one system for staging.

statistics – estimate; a collection of quantitative data.

stem cell rescue – a procedure in which stem cells (immature blood cells) are removed from the blood so they may be stimulated with growth factors in a lab in order to produce the growth of more stem cells; in a stem cell transplant, the patient then receives these new cells by transfusion.

steroid hormones – any of numerous compounds containing the carbon ring system of the sterols and including the sterols and various hormone and glycosides.

tofu – a soft cheese-like food that is made from a mixture of soybeans, a natural calcium-based coagulant and water.

transverse rectus abdominis myocutaneous or TRAM flap – one form of breast reconstruction which uses tissue from the lower abdominal wall to establish a breast mound on the chest.

vegetarian – a person who eats no meat; (a vegan eats no meat or animal products, including eggs, milk and even gelatin.)

web – the World Wide Web, a metaphor for information accessed on the Internet which is all linked together like a spider's Web.

website – the location of a collection of Web pages related to a specific subject; usually denoted by a unique domain name such as "cancer.org" or "oncolink.upenn.edu"

yoga – a Hindu philosophy teaching the suppression of all activity of the body, mind and will in order that the self may realize its distinction from them and attain liberation; a system of exercises for attaining bodily or mental control and well-being.

VISIT US ONLINE @ FIRSTAIDYOURSELF.ORG

Website Appendix

ACI's assessment of complementary and alternative treatments (http://www.cancer.org/alt_therapies/articles/index.html)
Air Care Alliance (http://www.aircareall.org/listings.htm)
AMA's doctor search page (http://www.ama-assn.org/iwcf/iwcfmgr206/aps?2331732074)
AMA's online publications page (http://www.ama-assn.org/med_link/peer.htm)
American Cancer Society (http://www.cancer.org/)
American Journalism Review Newslink (http://ajr.newslink.org/menu.html)
Association of Cancer Online Resources, Inc. (http://www.acor.org/)
Belle-Amie (http://www.belle-amie.com/)
Best Doctors (http://www.bestdoctors.com/)
BMT Support Online (http://users.aol.com/kendrabmt/bmtonli.htm)
BMT TALK (http://www.acor.org//listserv.html?to_do=interact&listname=BMT-TALK)
Bone Marrow Donors Worldwide (http://www.bmdw.org/)
Bone Marrow Foundation (http://www.bonemarrow.org/panic.html)
Bone Marrow Transplants (http://www.bmtnews.org/bmt/bmt.book/toc.html)
Bosom Buddies Breast Cancer Support, Inc (http://www.go-icons.com/bosombuddies.htm)
Bosom Buddies, Inc (http://www.bosombuddies.org/)
Breast Cancer Action (http://www.bcaction.org)
Breast Cancer Fund (http://www.breastcancerfund.org/)
Breast Cancer Information Services (http://trfn.clpgh.org/bcis/GeneralInfo/male.html)
ButterFly Image (http://www.bfi-ia.com/)
California Breast Cancer Treatment Fund (http://www.chpscc.org/bcedp/trtmnt.html)
Callanish Healing Retreats Society (http://www.callanish.org/)
Cancer Advocate's Caregiver Burnout (http://caregiver.com/march-april97/articles/burnout.html)
Cancer Advocate's Caregiver's Bill of Rights (http://caregiver.com/rights.html)
Cancer Care "Getting the Most Our of Your Health Insurance" (http://www.cancercare.org/clinical/insur13.htm)
Cancer Care "HMO's and Other Managed Care Plans" (http://www.cancercare.org/patients/hmos.htm)
Cancer Care "Information about 1986 COBRA Plans" (http://www.cancercare.org/patients/cobra.htm)
Cancer Care "Medical Insurance—a 'Hidden Crisis' for a Growing Number of Cancer Patients" (http://www.cancercare.org/patients/crisis.htm)
Cancer Care (http://www.cancercareinc.org/)

FIRST AID YOURSELF— ESSENTIAL BREAST CANCER WEBSITES

Cancer Care online support groups (http://www.cancercare.org/services/online3.htm)
Cancer Care's page on home care (http://www.cancercare.org/hhrd/hhrd_home.htm)
Cancer Hope Network (http://www.cancerhopenetwork.org/)
Cancer News (http://cancernews.com/quickload.htm)
Cancer-Free Connection (http://www.cancer-free.com/)
CancerBACUP's "Understanding Lymphedema" page (http://www.cancerbacup.org.uk/info/lymphedema.htm)
CancerCare (http://www.cancercare.org/)
CancerHelp online support groups (http://www.rwneill.com/cancerhelp.htm)
Cancerlist.org (http://www.cancerlinks.org)
Cancerlist/Cancerlinks (http://www.saklan.com/Cancerlist/) (http://www.acor.org/Cancerlist)
Care for the Caregiver (http://oncolink.upenn.edu/psychosocial/caregivers/care_caregiver.html)
CBR Environmental Endocrinology (http://www.tmc.tulane.edu/cbr/research/endocrinology.html)
CBR Environmental Estrogens and Other Hormones (http://www.tmc.tulane.edu/ECME/eehome/basics/estrogen/)
CBR Milestone page (http://www.tmc.tulane.edu/ECME/eehome/sources/milestones/)
Center for Mind-Body Medicine (http://www.healthy.net/cmbm)
CenterWatch (http://www.centerwatch.com/PROCAT12.HTM)
CenterWatch Drug List (http://www.centerwatch.com/drugs/DRUGLIST.HTM)
Charlotte Maxwell Complimentary Clinic (http://www.acupuncture.com/Referrals/Char.htm)
CNN cancer-related articles (http://cnn.com/HEALTH/cancer/)
CNN women's health page (http://cnn.com/HEALTH/indepth.health/womens.health/index.html)
Commonweal (http://www.commonweal.org/)
Corporate Angel Network (http://www.corpangelnetwork.org/)
Dallas Morning News "Learning to Live Again: AIDS patient embraces recovery after making peace with death"
    (http://www.aegis.com/news/dmn/1999/DN990101.html)
Doctors Guide to the Internet (http://www.pslgroup.com/docguide.htm)
Dr. Jeanne A. Petrek (http://www.mskcc.org/document/CN990610.htm)
Drug Infonet (http://www.druginfonet.com/hospital.htm)
Eastern Cooperative Oncology Group (http://ecog.dfci.harvard.edu/~ecogdba/general/active_prot.html)
ECRI Patient reference guide (http://www.hslc.org/emb/bc.txt)
Electric Library (http://www.elibrary.com/)

VISIT US ONLINE @ FIRSTAIDYOURSELF.ORG

Ernst Larsen's "Internet Cafe Guide" (http://www.netcafeguide.com/)
Free Internet Access (http://www.spinway.com)
Green Marketplace (http://www.greenmarketplace.com/)
Harmony Hill (http://www.harmonyhill.org/)
Harrie Meeuwissen's cybercafe list (http://usa.dedas.com/cybcaf.html)
HCFA phone numbers (http://www.hcfa.gov/regions/default.htm)
Health Care Choices (http://www.healthcarechoices.org/contact.htm)
Health Care Financing Administration (http://www.hcfa.gov/)
Health World Online (http://ww.healthy.net/welcome/index.asp)
Healthcare Users Group - HUG (http://www.bighug.com/)
Healthworks' Lymphedema FAQs (http://www.pblsh.com/Healthworks/lymfaqs.html)
High priority trials outside NCI (http://cancertrials.nci.nih.gov/)
IATP Endocrine Disrupter Resource Center (http://www.sustain.org/hcwh/main.htm)
Imperial Cancer Research Fund (http://www.lif.icnet.uk/research/factsheet/malebreast.html)
Inflammatory Breast Cancer (http://www.bestiary.com/ibc/)
Inspiration page (http://www.cancer-free.com/secrets.htm#psychology)
International Cancer Alliance for Research and Education (http://www.icare.org/)
Internet Appliance iOpener (http://www.netpliance.com)
Internet Drug Index (http://rxlist.com/)
JAMA's women's health page (http://www.ama-assn.org/special/womh/newsline/newsline.htm)
John Lester's hospital search page (http://neurowww2.mgh.harvard.edu/hospitalwebusa.html)
Keren Stronach's guide to transplants (http://comnet.org/nbmtlink/sg.html)
Komen Foundation (http://www.breastcancerinfo.com/bhealth/html/male_breast_cancer.asp)
Ladies First, Inc (http://www.wvi.com/~ladies1/)
Lilith Fair (http://www.lilithfair.com/)
Loansome Doc, to join (http://www.ncbi.nlm.nih.gov/PubMed/)
Lucy's Alternative Breast Implants (http://www.lucys.net/)
Madelon Hope's article, "What Can I Do About Hot Flashes And Night Sweats" (http://world.std.com/~susan207/flash.html)
Male Breast Cancer, Information Center (http://interact.withus.com/interact/mbc/)

An Original WebPointers™ Interactive Internet Guide © 2000 Hope Springs Press Inc

Male Breast Cancer, Department of Surgery, University of Iowa Hospitals and Clinics
(http://www.surgery.uiowa.edu/surgery/oncology/malebreastcancer.html)
Martindale's Health Science Guide's doctors/hospital search (http://sun2.lib.uci.edu/HSG/Pharmacy.html#DOCHOS)
Mayo Clinic's Health Oasis site for Women's Health (http://www.mayohealth.org/mayo/common/htm/womenpg2.htm)
Mothers & Others (http://www.mothers.org)
MSNBC breast cancer page (http://www.msnbc.com/news/BRCANCER_Front.asp)
National Alliance of Breast Cancer Organizations (http://www.nabco.org/facts/lymph.html)
National Association for Home Care (http://www.nahc.org/Consumer/coninfo.html)
National Bone Marrow Transplant Link (http://comnet.org/nbmtlink/)
National Cancer Institute (http://www.nci.nih.gov)
National Cancer Institute Overview (http://cancertrials.nci.nih.gov/NCI_CANCER_TRIALS/zones/TrialInfo/Finding/)
National Cancer Institute's CancerNet (http://cancernet.nci.nih.gov/clinpdq/canlit/breast.html)
National Cancer Institute's designated Cancer Centers (http://www.nci.nih.gov/cancercenters/centers1.htmv)
National Center for Complementary and Alternative Medicine (NCCAM) (http://nccam.nih.gov/)
National Foundation for Transplants (http://www.transplants.org/)
National Institutes of Health (http://www.nih.gov/)
National Library of Medicine's Medline (http://www.ncbi.nlm.nih.gov/Literature/index.html)
National Lymphedema Network (http://www.lymphnet.org/)
National Marrow Donor Program (http://www.marrow.org/2ndpage.html)
National Patient Air Transport Helpline (http://www.npath.org/index.a.html)
National Public Radio "The End of Life: Exploring Death in America" (http://www.npr.org/programs/death/)
National Race for the Cure (http://www.natl-race-for-the-cure.org/)
National Surgical Adjuvant Breast and Bowel Project (http://www.nsabp.pitt.edu/NSABP_Protocols.html)
National Transplant Assistance Fund (http://www.transplantfund.org/answer4.html)
NCI description of disease (http://rex.nci.nih.gov/PATIENTS/SITES_TYPES.html)
NCI disease summaries (http://cancernet.nci.nih.gov/pdq.htm)
NCI literature search (http://cnetdb.nci.nih.gov/cancerlit.shtml)
NCI-funded cancer center (http://cancertrials.nci.nih.gov/NCI_CANCER_TRIALS/zones/TrialInfo/Finding/centers/html/map.html)
Neutropenia (http://www.tirgan.com/leucpnia.htm)
New York Times (http://www.nytimes.com)
NewsEdge/NewsPage (www.newspage.com/)
North American Menopause Society (http://www.menopause.org/pfaq.htm)

OncoLink (http://www.oncolink.upenn.edu/disease/breast/treat/breast_recon2.html)
OncoLink's Caregiver Education Course (http://oncolink.upenn.edu/psychosocial/caregivers/)
Oncology Nursing Society (http://www.ons.org)
Organic Kitchen (http://www.organickitchen.com/)
P/S/L NuMedia Group's Complete Internet Medical Resource Doctor's Guide (http://www.pslgroup.com/dg/hospsite.htm)
Patient Advocate Foundation (http://www.patientadvocate.org)
Patient Advocates (http://www.patientadvocacy.org)
Patrick Hudson's (http://www.phudson.com/breastrecon.html)
Physician's Desk Reference Family Guide to Women's Health (http://www.healthsquare.com/pdrfg/wh/chapters/wh1ch28.htm)
Precision Therapeutics in Pittsburgh, Pennsylvania (http://www.ptilabs.com)
Public Internet access locations (http://cybercaptive.com/pia.shtml)
P\S\L Consulting Group Inc.'s Doctor's Guide—Menopause Information and Resources (http://www.pslgroup.com/MENOPAUSE.HTM)
Quackwatch (http://www.quackwatch.com)
Radiation Therapy Oncology Group (http://www.rtog.org/)
Rational Therapeutics Cancer Laboratories (http://www.rational-t.com/index.html)
Smith Farm Center for the Healing Arts (http://www.smithfarm.com/)
Southwest Oncology Group (http://www.oo.saci.org/Breast3.html)
Steve Dunn on Chemosensitivity testing (http://www.cancerguide.org/unconv_conv.html)
Steve Dunn's Cancer Guide (http://www.cancerguide.org/)
Steve Dunn's write-up of clinical trials (http://www.cancerguide.org/clinical_trials.html)
Studio International (http://studiohair.net)
Susan G. Komen Breast Cancer Foundation (http://www.breastcancerinfo.com)
The Apothecary (http://www.intr.net/apothecary/index.html)
Ting-Sha Cancer Help Program (http://www.amacord.com/tingsha/index.html)
Tirgan Oncology Associates (http://www.tirgan.com/)
Trials at the Bethesda, Maryland Campus (http://www-dcs.nci.nih.gov/clin_trials/)
University of Chicago Breast Cancer Comprehensive Center (http://phoenicia.bsd.uchicago.edu/index.cgi/175005883)
University of Iowa Plastic Surgery page (http://www.surgery.uiowa.edu:80/surgery/plastic/brecon.html)
University of Pennsylvania's OncoLink (http://www.oncolink.upenn.edu/clinical_trials/protocols.html)
University of Pennsylvania's OncoLink cancer site (http://oncolink.upenn.edu/)

University of Texas MD Anderson Cancer Center (http://www.mdanderson.org/)
University of Texas's Center for Alternative Medicine Research in Cancer (UTCAM) (http://www.sph.uth.tmc.edu/utcam/)
Updates (http://cancertrials.nci.nih.gov/NCI_CANCER_TRIALS/zones/PressInfo/updates.html)
USA TODAY (http://www.usatoday.com)
Victorian Order of Nurses (http://www.von.ca/)
Washington Post (http://www.washingtonpost.com)
When The Woman You Love Has Breast Cancer (http://www.y-me.org/partner.html)
Women's Environment and Development Organization (http://www.wedo.org)
WRI's "Environmental Influences on Breast Cancer Risks" (http://www.wri.org/health/med-e-br.html)
WRI's Business and Environment Resources Worldwide page (http://www.wri.org/meb/links.html)
WRI's Health and Environment page (http://www.wri.org/health/)
WWF Endocrine Disruptors page (http://worldwildlife.org/toxics/progareas/ed/index.htm)
Y-ME National Breast Cancer Organization (http://www.yme.org/)
Yahoo!'s Breast Cancer coverage (http://headlines.yahoo.com/Full_Coverage/Tech/Breast_Cancer)
Yahoo!'s organic food page (http://dir.yahoo.com/Business_and_Economy/Companies/Food/Natural_Organic/)
You Are Not Alone (YANA) (http://www.yana.org/)
You Are Not Alone (YANA) medical records (http://www.yana.org/medicalrecords.htm)

Additional Resources

Information available on the Internet is expanding without apparent limits.

The number of pages on the World Wide Web passed the billion mark in December, 1999. New pages are being added at an estimated rate of three million per day. No search engine claims to have a complete catalog of all the Webpages available and no one has offered any hope—or evidence—that the search engines will one day catch up.

The following online resources either appeared on the Web after author Betsy Dance completed her narrative or were not found during her many, many attempts to find information for her friend Ellen. They are presented here to help you with your searches.

Some, like ibc survivor Alexandra Andrews's *Cancer Links*, (see p. 22) which went online on February 14, 1999 have continued to evolve and improve since first visited. If you were asked to name the three most helpful breast cancer Websites online in mid-2000 this would be a definite; the other two would be hard to nail down unless you had also discovered her *cancerlynx.org* and *cancerlinks.com* which was launched in mid-May, 2000 with the promise of being "cancerlinks.org with an attitude."

If you visit no other Website, you owe it to yourself to go to *Cancer Link's Web Tutorial Program* developed by Andrews, Annamarie Baldassari and Bob Gill in November of 1999. This excellent teaching tool explains not only how to find information online but gives simple illustrations of exactly what your computer screen will look like as you take each step. Cancer Links is available in Spanish and is also accessible to the blind and visually impaired.

This list is not exhaustive. Nor can it be. As the Web continues to evolve, more valuable sites will appear, less valuable ones will disappear. It is the nature of the value of information.

As always, it is important to remember that a free market in information puts all the responsibility for evaluating content on you the reader. Be forewarned. Some information may be erroneous. Some may have been accurate once, but is no longer. Seek corroboration. Trust known sources. Be skeptical of claims that appear to good to be true. Test all assumptions. Get second opinions.

And when you find something very, very good, pass it on.

We are always interested to learn of new Websites and will, from time to time, update this list for eBook users. Feedback is welcome.

Email Publisher@firstaidyourself.org

FIRST AID YOURSELF— ESSENTIAL BREAST CANCER WEBSITES

American Academy of Family Physicians (http://www.familydoctor.org)
American Cancer Society's Breast Cancer Network (http://www2.cancer.org/bcn.htm)
American College of Obstetricians and Gynecologists (http://www.acog.org)
American College of Radiology (http://www.radiologyinfo.org)
American Institute for Cancer Research (http://www.aicr.org)
American Medical Women's Association (http://www.amwa-doc.org)
American Society of Clinical Oncology (http://www.asco.org)
AstraZeneca Healthcare Foundation (http://www.astrazeneca.com)
Breast Cancer Information Center (http://www.feminist.org/other/bc/bchome.html)
Breast Cancer in The Family, by Leah deRoulet (http://www1.mightywords.com/asp/bookinfo/bookinfo.asp?theisbn=EB00005577)
Breast Doc (http://www.breastdoc.com)
Breast Link Breast Cancer Care & Research Fund (http://www.breastlink.com)
Cancer Facts (http://www.cancerfacts.com)
Cancer Links (http://www.cancerlinks.org)
Cancer Links —with an attitude (http://www.cancerlinks.com)
Cancer Lynx (http://www.cancerlynx.com)
CancerNet (http://cancernet.nci.nih.gov)
Cancer Page (http://www.cancerpage.com)
Cancer Research Foundation of America (http://www.crfa.org)
Cancer Research Institute (http://www.cancerresearch.org)
Cancer Supportive Care (http://www.cancersupportivecare.com)
CanHelp (http://www.canhelp.com)
Centers for Disease Control and Prevention (http://www.cdc.gov/cancer)
Chemocare (http://www.cancerhopenetwork.org)
Continuum Health Partners' Guide to Breast Cancer (http://www.wehealny.org/services/breast/index.html)
Disease, Disorders and Related Topics (http://www.mic.ki.se/Diseases))
Entre Mujeres *[Spanish site]* (http://www.cancerlinks.com/Mujeres/mujeres.html)
Force: Facing Our Risk of Cancer Empowered (http://www.facingourrisk.org)
General Cancer News (http://www.cancernnews.com/cancernews.htm)
Hardin MD—Hardin Meta Directory of Internet Health Sources (http://www.lib.uiowa.edu/hardin/md/index.html)
Healthscope (http://www.healthscope.org)

Home Care Guide for Advanced Cancer (http://www.acponline.org/public/homecare)
Kidscope (http://www.kidscope.org/kids.html)
Living Beyond Breast Cancer (http://www.lbbc.org)
Mammacare (http://www.mammacare.com)
Mary-Helen Mautner Project for Lesbians with cancer (http://www.mautnerproject.org)
Medline (http://www.healthgate.com)
MedWebPlus—Health Science Information Index (http://www.medwebplus.com)
National Cancer Research Foundation (http://www.crfa.org)
National Action Plan on Breast Cancer (http://www.napbc.org)
National Breast Cancer Resource List (http://www.natlbcc.org)
National Breast Cancer Awareness Month (http://www.nbcam.com)
National Cancer Database (http://www.facs.org/about_college/acsdept/cancer_dept/programs/ncdb/ncdb.html)
National Medical Association (http://www.nmanet.org)
Oncology Nursing Society (http://www.ons.org/xp6/ONS/Login/Patients_Consumers.xml)
Public Health Institute's Breast Cancer Answers (http://www.canceranswers.org)
SusanLoveMd (http://www.susanlovemd.com)
Thehealthchannel.com (http://www.the healthchannel.com)
Wellness Community (http://www.twc-chat.org)
WIN Against Breast Cancer (http://www.winabc.org)
Women's Cancer Resource Center (http://www.wcrc.org)
Womens Cancer Scripts (http://www.cancerscripts.org)

Examining Your Own Breasts

A growing number of Websites offer tips and techniques for Breast Self Examination (BSE). The following is the editors' choice for the most straightforward explanation of this important and simple technique which is the first line of defence for breast health. It is written by Dr. Deborah Axelrod, Chief of the Breast Center at St. Vincent's Comprehensive Cancer Center in New York City and reprinted, by special permission, from her Website — http://www.breastdoc.com

*Dr. Axelrod is co-author, with Rosie O'Donnell and Tracy Chutorian Semler, of "**Bosom Buddies**, Lessons and Laughter on Breast Health and Cancer" Warner Books; ISBN: 0446676209*

Figure 1

By Deborah Axelrod, MD, FACS

There are several techniques, including one in which you go round and round the breasts in a circular motion, (see Fig. 1) and another in which you do a series of up-and-down strip searches of the breast and pie-shaped wedges (see Fig. 2). I strongly prefer the up-and-down (vertical) strip search method, (see Fig. 3) as it tends to cover all of the breast tissue. With the circular method, it's easier to miss a ring of breast tissue as you're going round and round.

The Mammacare BSE learning system (www.mammacare.com) is a very useful breast model that contains several simulated breast tumors and other lumps. You can use the model to practice the breast self-exam and to get a better idea of what to feel inside the breast.

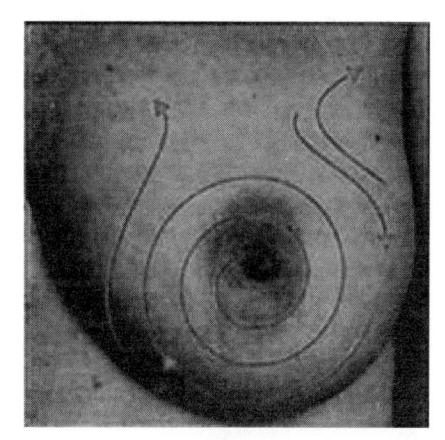

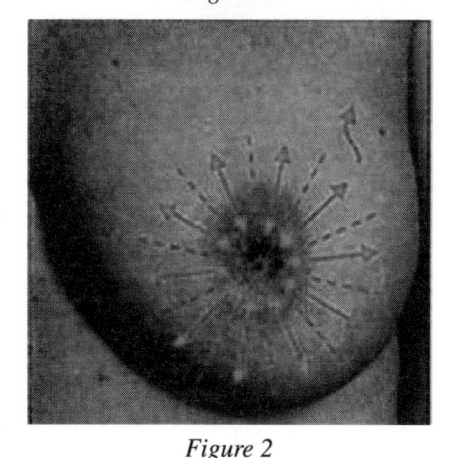

Figure 2

© 2000 Deborah Axelrod, M.D. Breast Doc.com. All Rights Reserved

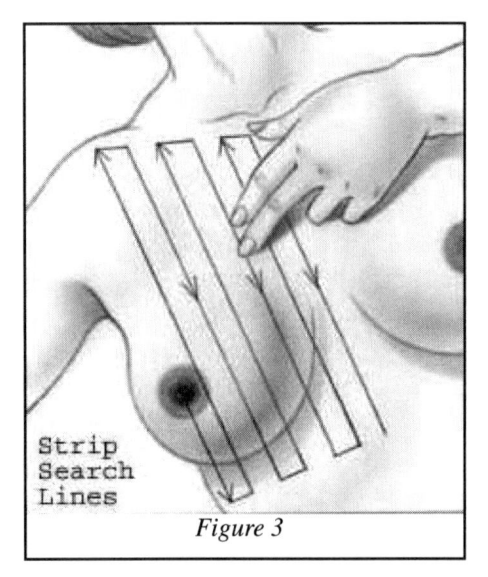

I sometimes give a small test breast model (with two masses inside) to women in my office. It can be purchased though Health Edco® in Waco, Texas. Health Edco® 1-800-299-3366 x 295.

There are two key concepts involved in the proper use of this method of breast self-exam. The first one involves using three different levels of pressure when feeling the breasts (see Fig. 4). The idea is to check the breast at various depths, rather than doing one simple check in which you try to push all the way down inside the breast.

Figure 3

How To Use Your Fingers

Using the pads of your fingers, (see Fig 5) first apply light pressure to the breast, as you are checking the area just slightly underneath the breast skin's surface. Next, apply medium pressure to the breast, checking about midway inside the breast. And finally, apply deep pressure,

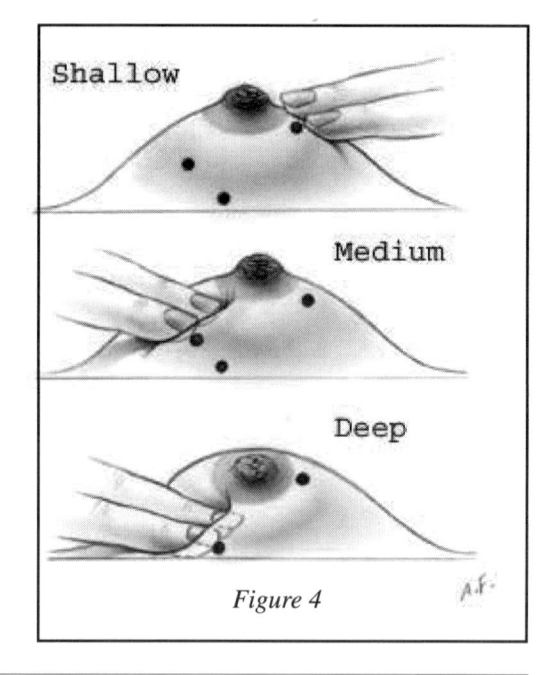

Figure 4

© 2000 Deborah Axelrod, M.D. Breast Doc.com. All Rights Reserved

feeling for the area deepest in the breast. You should use these three pressures as you examine your breasts.

The second critical concept in doing the breast self-exam is to cover all of your breast tissue; that tissue can cover a lot more ground than most women realize. Breast tissue often extends up to the collarbone; down to the rib cage or even below the rib cage and bra line; and all the way to each underarm. Your self-exam should cover this landscape as well. And most important, do not allow your fingers to stop or lift away from your breast at any point in the middle of the exam. Here's what to do:

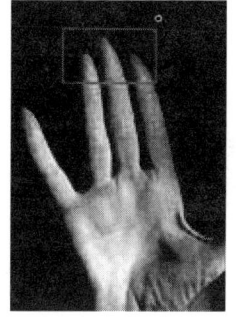

Lie on your side, but twist back a bit so your breast falls as flat as possible on your chest, rather than hanging down toward the floor (see Fig. 6). This helps you to cover more surface area and allows you to apply firm pressure against a hard surface. Now you can begin your "strip search" of the breast. Do your light, medium, and deep presses in straight lines moving in vertical lines from your collarbone down below your bra line and covering the area from the armpit to the breastbone. Use the left arm to check the right breast and vice versa. You might want to use

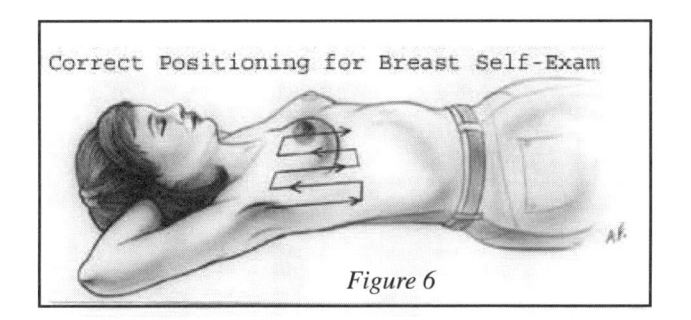

Figure 5

Figure 6

© 2000 Deborah Axelrod, M.D. Breast Doc.com. All Rights Reserved

lotion or powder to help you move over the breast smoothly. Do not squeeze the nipples. If you notice a discharge, bring this to the attention of your doctor.

Examine breasts one at a time, and examine both breasts every time. And do the exam every month. With time, you will become intimately familiar with the architecture of your breasts, and well equipped to tell your doctor about any new changes in them. If you feel a new potential "abnormality," check the other breast in the same region to see if it's symmetrical.

When to Do Your Self-Exam

It's useful to do the breast self-exam at the same time each month, because the breasts tend to change (as a result of changing hormones) throughout a woman's monthly cycle. If you have a regular menstrual cycle, then the best time to do the breast self-exam is about seven to ten days after your period begins each month. At this time, your breasts are the least lumpy and the least tender to the touch.

If you don't have regular monthly periods, then try to do your breast self-exam on the same day each month—for example, on the first of every month, the day you pay your monthly bills, your bridge game, or something else you won't forget.

Most women's breasts have lots of bumpy or nodular areas in them. Only young girls' breasts are perfectly smooth. The goal in checking your breasts is to find dominant lumps—something that stands out and that is not symmetrical with the

© 2000 Deborah Axelrod, M.D. Breast Doc.com. All Rights Reserved

other breast. Symmetry is very important: if you find the same lump on the other breast, it's usually normal.

Search for lumps that are hard, irregular in shape, not painful, and not mobile (i.e., something that's attached to the skin or muscle and that doesn't move). These can be (but aren't always) problem signs, and should be brought to your doctor's attention. The lump can be in the breast area, under the arm, or anywhere else in the region. Also, if such a lump is associated with a change on the skin of your breast, tell your doctor.

On the contrary, lumps that are mobile, smooth, painful, and unattached are generally nothing to worry about, but always need investigation. Certainly painful lumps can be cancerous. Always tell your doctor of a new lump.

Finally, remember that breast tumors appear in areas other than the breast itself. Breast tissue can extend all the way over to the underarm; up to the collarbone; and down to the rib cage.

The bottom line is, you can't be perfect. Even doctors trained in evaluating breast lumps are wrong up to 30 percent of the time when making judgments about what they feel in their patients' breasts. You can't expect much more of yourself.

Do the best you can—and bring anything suspicious to your doctor's attention.

© 2000 Deborah Axelrod, M.D. Breast Doc.com. All Rights Reserved

Acronyms

ACA — Air Care Alliance
ACI — American Cancer Institute
ACOR — Association of Cancer Online Resources
ACS — American Cancer Society
AIDS — Auto Immune Deficiency
AMA — American Medical Association
AOL — America OnLine
BBBCSI — Bosom Buddies Breast Cancer Support, Inc.
BCIS — Breast Cancer Information Services
BMT — Bone Marrow Transplant
CBCTF — California Breast Cancer Treatment Fund
CBR — Center for Bioenvironmental Research
CCHP — Commonweal Cancer Help Program
CNN — Cable News Network
ECRI — Emergency Care Research Institute
HCFA — Health Care Financing Administration
HMO — Health Maintenance Organization
IATP — Endocrine Disrupter Resource Center
IATP — Institute for Agriculture and Trade Policy
ICARE — International Cancer Alliance for Research and Education
ICRF — Imperial Cancer Research Fund

JAMA — Journal of the American Medical Association
MMA — Mercy Medial Airlift
MSNBC — MicroSoft National Broadcasting Network
NABCO — National Alliance of Breast Cancer Organizations
NCPATS — National Charitable Patient Air Transportation System
NFT — National Foundation for Transplants
NIH — National Institutes of Health
NLN — National Lymphedema Network
NMDP — National Marrow Donor Program
NPATH — National Patient Air Transport Helpline
NPR — National Public Radio
NSABP — National Surgical Adjuvant Breast and Bowel Project
NTAF — National Transplant Assistance Fund
OTA — Office of Technology Assessment
POPS — Persistent Organic Pollutants
TBCF — The Breast Cancer Fund
WWF — World Wildlife Fund
YANA — You Are Not Alone

Index

Abdomen, 68
Abnormality, 97
Abstracts, 20, 33, 95
Academy of Motion Picture Arts, 73
ACA—Air Care Alliance, 70-71
ACS—American Cancer Society, 20
Action, A Call To, 12, 91
Acupuncture, 62-63, 95-96
Adjuvant, 31, 95
Adrenal, 97
Adriamycin, 61, 95
Advocacy, 22, 69, 90-91
Ailments, 97
Air Care Alliance, 70-71
Alley, Dr. Katherine, 42
Allogenic, 76, 95
Alone, You Are Not, (YANA), 23, 52-53
Alternative Breast Implants, 73
Alternative, 9, 21, 39, 44-47, 55, 73, 96
American Cancer Society, 20-21
American Journalism Review, 49
American Medical Association, 27, 33
Amputation, 74, 98
Anderson Cancer Center, 26-27
Andrews, Alexandra, 22, 84
Anthracycline, 95
Anti-cancer, 36
Antibiotic, 95
Antioxidant, 37, 45, 96
Apologetic, 82

Apothecary, 38-39
Apron, 40
Areola, 72
Assessment, 20-21, 55
Atcom-Iport Cyberbooths, 25
Autologous, 95
Axelrod, Deborah, 88

Bacteriology, 99
Baldness, 40
Ballooning, 74
Barrett, Dr. Stephen, 47
BBBCSI—Bosom Buddies Breast Cancer Support, Inc., 74
BCIS—Breast Cancer Information Services, 85
Belle-Amie, 72-73
Best Doctors, 26-27
Bevin, Pete, 34
Bioenvironmental, 86
Blum, Diane S., 52
BMT—Bone Marrow Transplant, 76
Bone Marrow, 10, 29, 34, 60, 76-79, 95, 97, 99
Bosom Buddies Breast Cancer Support, (BBBCSI), 74
Boston Globe, 49, 51
Boston University, 60
Boston, 49, 51, 60
Bowel Project, 31

Bowel, 31
Brainchild, 12, 66
Branch, 99
Breast Cancer
  Action, 90-91
  Environmental Causes of, 91
  Fund, 63, 90-91
  Information Services, 85
  Male, 10, 84-85
  Metastatic, 76
  Patients, A Companion Guide for, 77
  Risks, 88-89
  Treatment, 32, 63
Bristol-Myers Squibb, 83
Brown, Janie, 57
Brown, Richard K. J., 50
Burdock root, 46, 97
Burzynski, Stanislaw R., 44

C-section, 82
Caisse, Rene, 97
California Breast Cancer Treatment Fund, (CBCTF), 63
Callanish Healing Retreats Society, 57
Cancer
  Advocate, 59
  Center, 26-27, 31, 44, 52, 59
  Guide, 22-23
  Help Program, 55-57
  Hope Network, 43
  News, 50-51

Prevention Campaign, 91
Therapy Review, 21
CancerCare, 35, 53, 63, 65
CancerHelp, 35
Cancerlinks, 22-23, 84
Cancerlit, 21
CancerNet, 21, 33
Cancernews, 51
Cancertrials, 31
Carcinogens, 10, 88-89, 96
Carcinoma, 20, 98
Caregiver Burnout, 59
Caregiver, 58-59
Carnegie Science Center, 36
Carson, Rachel, 89
CBCTF—California Breast Cancer Treatment Fund, 63
CCHP—Commonweal Cancer Help Program, 55
Center for Bioenvironmental Research, 86
CenterWatch, 27, 61
Charlotte Maxwell Complimentary Clinic, 62-63
Chemical-free, 39
CHEMOcare, 43
ChemoFxAssay, 36
Chemotherapy, 21, 23, 34-36, 38, 42, 44-46, 59-61, 64, 66, 68, 72, 76, 82, 92, 95-99
Chicago Tribune, 49
Chicago, 49, 55, 58-59, 68-69

Child Health Insurance Program, 52
Child, Julia, 29
Citrate, 97
City of Hope National Medical Center, 29
Clearinghouse, 32, 75, 79
Climb Against The Odds, 91
Clomiphene, 97
Clothes, 64, 74
Clothing, 72
Club Disney, 25
COBRA Plans, 53
Coenzyme Q10, 45
Coleman, Barbara Smith, 56
Coleman, Douglas, 78
Colon, 44, 80
Commonweal Cancer Help Program, (CCHP), 55
Complementary Medicine, 38, 44, 46-47, 55
Complete Internet Medical Resource Doctor, 26-27
Complication, 60, 74, 98
Compounds, 96, 99
Comprehensive Cancer Database, 20
Comprehensive Care Conference, 44
Contaminants, 88-90
Corporate Angel Network, 70-71
Cortex, 97
Cyberbooths, 25
Cybercafe Search Engine, 25

Dalby, Sabra, 80
Dallas Morning News, 81
Dana Farber Cancer Institute, 52
Dandelion, 66
Davenport-Ennis, Nancy, 53
Davis, Dr. Devra Lee, 88
Desk Reference Family Guide, 83
Diagnostic Radiology, 50
Diarrhea, 21, 96
Dioxin, 89, 96, 99
Disrupter Information, 87
Disrupters, 86-87, 96
Division of Cancer Treatment, 44
Donors Worldwide, 79
Dose-dense, 34, 66, 96
Double-mastectomy, 29
Doxorubicin, 61, 95
Drug Infonet, 27

Ecosystem Health, 88
ECRI—Emergency Care Research Institute, 76
Electric Library, 49
Emergency Care Research Institute, (ECRI), 76
Emergency Volunteer Aircorps, 71
End of Life, 81
Endocrinology, 86-87
Endocrinology, 86-87
Essiac tea, 46, 97
Estrogen, 19, 86-88, 97
Estrogens, 10, 86-88, 99

Exploring Death, 81

F.K., 32, 41, 54-55, 58-59
Fair, Dr. William R., 44
Falsies, 72
Fatigue, 60
Feminine, 40-41, 68
Fertility, 18-19, 87, 97
Flu, 61

Gelatin, 100
Georgetown, 26, 56
Glycosides, 99
Gonadotropic, 97
Gordon, James S., 44
Goulet, Robert, 29
Grayson
 Ellen Lea Hickey, 17-128
 Roger, 18, 24, 38-39, 41, 50, 52, 54, 59-60, 61, 64-65, 69, 70, 82, 87, 90, 92
 Stafford Olivia Sommers, 17-19, 33, 40-41, 52, 54, 60-61, 64, 66-67, 70, 74, 81-82, 87, 90
Grimmel, Cheryl, 53
GTE Cyberbooths, 25
Gynecomastia, 84, 97

Hælth, 44
Hair, 9, 40-41, 54, 81-82
Hankins, Dr. David, 21
Harmony Hill, 57
Harvard Medical School, 37

Hawaii Cancer Help Retreats, 57
HCFA—Health Care Financing Administration, 52
Healing Arts, 56-57
Health Care Financing Administration, (HCFA), 52-53
Health Insurance Resources Center, 53
Health Oasis, 83
Health Science Guide, 27
Health World Online, 45
Healthworks, 75
Healthy Travel, 45
Hendricks, Dr. Carolyn, 26
Herbal, 44-46, 83
Herbs, 67, 97
Hetrick, Virginia, 23, 52
Hidden Crisis, 53
High-Dose Chemotherapy, 23, 76, 96-97
Hindu, 100
Hollywood, 72
Homeopathy, 62
Hope, Madelon, 83
Hormones, 18, 86-87, 96-99
Hospice Locator, 65
Hot Flashes And Night Sweats, 83
Hudis, Dr. Clifford, 26
Hudson, Patrick, 69

IATP—Endocrine Disrupter Resource Center, 87

IATP—Institute for Agriculture and Trade Policy, 87
ICARE—International Cancer Alliance for Research and Education, 21
Iceland, 21, 97
ICRF—Imperial Cancer Research Fund, 85
Immediate Help, 65
Immunology-based, 36, 97
Imperial Cancer Research Fund, ICRF, 85
Inflammatory Breast Cancer, 19-20, 23, 26, 30, 32, 35-36, 92, 97
Information Center, 84-85
Insurance, 23, 37, 50, 52-53, 62-63, 71-72, 74, 78
International Cancer Alliance, 21
Internet Cafe Guide, 24-25
Internet Drug Index, 61

Jackson Hole, WY, 36
JAMA—Journal of the American Medical Association, 33
Johns Hopkins Medical School, 21
Journal of Clinical Oncology, 33
Journal of the American Medical Association, 33

Kanzler, Clay, 80
Kashi, 39, 98
Kinko's, 25
Kitchen Table Wisdom, 56

Komen, Susan G., Breast Cancer Foundation, 62-63, 84, 91
Ladies First, 73
Lancet, The, 33
Landro, Laura, 26
Language of Cancer, 90
Largest On-Line Salon, 40
Larsen, Ernst, 24-25
Latissimus, 68, 98
Lester, 27
Lethargic, 60
Leukemia, 26, 98
Leukocytes, 98
Lichen, 97
Life-sustaining, 66
Life-threatening, 42, 64, 85, 98
Lilith Fair, 91
Lilly, Eli, 83
Limb, Ballooning, 74
Livingston Wheeler Clinic, 42
Loansome Doc, 33
Longworth, Alice Roosevelt, 29
Los Angeles Times, 49
Los Angeles, CA, 49, 73
Lump, 84, 97
Lymphatic, 74-75, 97
Lymphedema Action Plan, 74
Lymphedema FAQs, 75
Lymphedema Prevention, 74

Mammogram, 12, 84
Managed Care Plans, 52-53

Marron, Tom, 29
Marrow Transplant Newsletter, 77
Martin, Andrea, 91
Massachusetts General Hospital, 27, 37
Massage, 55-56, 62
Mastectomies, 72
Mastitis, 19, 98
Maxwell, Charlotte, 62-63
Mayo Clinic, 83
Medicaid, 52
Medicare, 52
Medicine, Alternative, 46-47
Medline, 32-33
Meeuwissen, Harrie, 25
Mega-doses, 18
Melanoma, 29, 80, 98
Memorial Sloan-Kettering Cancer Center, 26, 44, 52
Menopause, 10, 82-83, 97-98
Mercy Medical Airlift Charitable Air Transportation, 71
Miami Herald, 49
Milestone, 87
Milken, Michael, 29
Mind-Body Medicine, 44-45, 51
Mind-body, 44-45, 51, 98
Mitochondrial, 96
MMA, (Mercy Medical Airlift), 71
Myocutaneous, 68, 100

NABCO—National Alliance of Breast Cancer Organizations, 75

Nagourney, Dr. Robert, 37
Nashville, TN, 36
National
  Alliance of Breast Cancer Organizations, (NABCO), 75
  Bone Marrow Transplant Link, 76-77
  Charitable Patient Air Transportation System, (NCPATS), 71
  Legal Resource Network, 53
  Library of Medicine, 30-33
  Lymphedema Network, 74-75
  Managed Care Resource Network, 53
  Marrow Donor Program, 78-79
  Patient Air Transport Helpline, 71
  Public Radio, 81
  Surgical Adjuvant Breast and Bowel Project, 31
  Transplant Assistance Fund, 78-79
Natural Healing, 44
Nausea, 20, 95, 98
NCPATS—National Charitable Patient Air Transportation System, 71
Nearly Me, 73
Neuro-oncology, 37
Neutropenia, 60-61, 98
New England Journal of Medicine, 33
New York Times, 48-49
NewsPage, 51
NFT—National Foundation for Transplants, 78
NIH—National Institutes of Health, 20-21

NLN—National Lymphedema Network, 75
Nodes, 74, 97-98
North American Menopause Society, 83
NPATH—National Patient Air Transport Helpline, 71
NTAF—National Transplant Assistance Fund, 78
Nurses, 60, 65
Nursing, 19, 60, 77
Nutritional, 44, 50
Nutritionist, 38

O'Toole, Carol, 40, 42
Oakland, CA, 62
OB-GYN, 18
Office of Technology Assessment, (OTA), 55
Oncologists, 28, 32, 42, 46
Oncology Nursing Society, 77
Oncology, 27-29, 33, 35, 44, 50, 60-61, 77, 85
Online Doctor Finder, 27
Organ Transplant Fund, 78
Organic Kitchen, 39
Organic, 38-39, 50, 65, 89, 96, 98-99
Organically-grown, 39
Organics, 39
Osborne, Michael P., 88
Osteopathy, 95

OTA—Office of Technology Assessment, 55

Panic When Coverage Is Denied, 78
Parton, Dolly, 40
Pathologists, 97
Patients-in-need, 79
Peabody, Annie, 80
Pesticides, 38-39, 96, 98
Petrek, Dr. Jeanne A., 68-69
Phthalates, 99
Physicians, 26, 31, 75, 79
Phytoestrogens, 86, 99
Pittsburgh Breast Care Test Coalition, 85
Pittsburgh, PA, 36, 85
Pituitary, 97
Plastic Surgery, 68-69
Point Reyes, CA, 56
Pollution, 88-89
Polyvinylchloride, 99
Post-mastectomy, 73-74, 98
Pregnancy, 68, 82, 95
Pregnant, 18-19, 82
Progesterone, 97
Prospect of Death, 10, 59, 80-81
Prosthesis, 69, 72
Protocol, 26, 34, 96, 99
Puberty, 82-83
Public Internet, 25
PubMed, 32-33

Quackwatch, 47

Radiology, 50
Rainbow Organics, 39
Raloxifene, 90
Rational Therapeutics Cancer Laboratories, 37
Reconstruction, 68-69, 97, 100
Rectus, 68, 100
Remedies, 44-45, 83
Remen, Dr. Rachel Naomi, 56
Remission, 28, 30, 99
Reproductive, 86, 88-89
Researchers, 12-13, 31, 33-34, 88
Researching Clinical Trials, 9, 30
Researching, 9, 30, 48
Resources, Association of Cancer Online (ACOR), 34-35
Retreats, 56-57
Reuters, 51
Rhubarb, 46, 97
Robertson, Dave, 45
Rosenberg, Irv, 38, 42

Schodde, Gretchen, 57
Schwarzkopf, Norman, 29
Scott-Conner, Dr. Carol, 84
Sexuality, 82-83
Silent Spring, 89
Silicone, 68, 73
Sky Links, 25
Smith Farm Cancer Help Program, 56

Sorrel, 46, 97
South Africa, 24
Soy, 38-39
Soybeans, 100
Specialty Research Centers, 46
Sri Lanka, 24
Standard-Bearers, 20
Starpoint, 55
Steingraber, Sandra, 89
Stimulant, 45
Stomach, 92, 98
Streep, Meryl, 89
Stress, 65, 68, 78
Stressbusters, 23
Stresses, 88, 92
Strohecker, James, 45
Stronach, Keren, 76-77
Studio International, 40-41
Sudan, 64
Sugar, 38
Supportive Care Summaries, 20
Survival, 29-30, 84-85

Taking Control of Your Fight Against Cancer, 26
Tamoxifen, 90
TBCF—The Breast Cancer Fund, 90
Telang, Nitin T., 88
Temple, LuAnne, 73
Thiadens, Saskia R. J., 75
Thielbar, Janice M., 72
Tiegs, Cheryl, 40

Ting-Sha Institute, 56
Tirgan Oncology Associates, 60-61
Tirgan, M. Hossein, 60
Tissues, 97-98
Tofu, 39, 64, 100
Tomato, 46
Touchnet Kiosks, 25
Toxins, 38, 88-89
Transfusion, 95, 99
Transplant, (BMT), 76
Transportation, 63, 70-71
Tufts University, 73
Tulane, Bioenvironmental Research of, 86

UCLA, 73
Unconventional Cancer Treatments, 55
United Nations Environment Program Treaty Process, 89
University
   Hospital, 26, 29
   of Chicago, Breast Cancer Comprehensive Center, 68-69
   of Iowa, 68-69, 84-85
   of Pittsburgh Medical Center, 36
   of Texas MD Anderson Cancer Center, 26-27
Urologic Oncology, Department of, 44
Use of Compression Pumps, 74

Vanderbilt Univ. Medical School, 21
Veach, Virginia, 57
Vegetarian Direct, 39

Vegetarian, 39, 54-55, 100
Victorian Order of Nurses, 65
Vitamins, 50
Walbridge, Sally, 91
Wall Street Journal, 26
Washington Post, 48-49
Weinstein, Mickey, 38
Welch, Raquel, 40
Wigs, 40
Wittes, Robert E., 44
Wolfe, Menya, 34
Worden, Bill, 71
Working, 22, 52, 66, 91
World Resources Institute, 88
WWF Endocrine Disrupters, 87
WWF—World Wildlife Fund, 87

Xavier Universities, 86

YANA—You Are Not Alone, 23, 52-53

Acknowledgments

My thanks to Jack McShea and Clarisa Hooper for saving my writing life in Montana by patiently and generously repairing my lemon computer, and to Peter Krogh for trying to do the same in Washington. To Kate, who helped me leave Washington. To Brian Haave, who made it possible. To all the people along the way from New Mexico to Montana, (especially Kate Bermingham; Trula and Percy Cooper; Pam and Jim Barlow;) who gave me hearth and home that was not a Motel 6. And to Lily Whiteman, who has been there every inch of the way—emailing me Internet sites, letting me stay in her apartment when I have since visited Ellen, and making life spirited and carefree when it has been nothing of the sort.

Thanks to Robin Lind and Kitty Williams for their longstanding and extensive understanding of friendship, for their vision and for their skills and talents, without which this would not be a book.

I am also indebted to many people along the way who have adopted this book during its birthing process and taken on, unbidden, the role of literary adjuvant. Some I have never met. Some have moved so discreetly and anonymously I know only their good works. But among those who must be counted among this book's godparents, I name Alice Acheson, Deborah Axelrod, Ernie Bodai, Penelope deBordenave Saffer, Currie Smith, Peter Stalker, Jon Russell, and Jim Wilson. Thank you.

VISIT US ONLINE @ FIRSTAIDYOURSELF.ORG

Betsy Dance

Betsy Dance was graduated from the University of Virginia and earned an MA in creative writing from Johns Hopkins University. Her work has appeared in such national publications as The Washington Post, Reader's Digest, and The New Yorker.

She grew up in Grosse Pointe, Michigan with her friend Ellen Lea Hickey Grayson, and returned to her homestate in 1999 to found LocalMotion, a non-profit organization dedicated to raising awareness of the links between environmental toxins and cancer.

First Aid Yourself was first published in an eBook edition in June, 2000. The printed edition was published to coincide with October Breast Cancer Awareness Month and is available from fine bookstores everywhere. It may also be ordered online from FirstAidYourself.org where special pricing will be offered for groups and organizations that wish to purchase in quantity for further fund-raising activities.

Purchasers of the printed book are entitled to download the eBook edition at no additional charge; if you purchased the eBook edition online you may receive the companion printed edition for only the cost of shipping and handling.

Please register at http://www.firstaidyourself.org.

The design for First Aid Yourself, Essential Breast Cancer Websites, reflects the influence of Master Typographer Jan Tschichold. The horizontal proportions were chosen to offer the best onscreen presentation for the companion eBook edition which is published in Adobe System's Portable Document Format. Text is typeset in Gill Sans, headlines in Giovanni Book.

Online encryption and distribution of the eBook edition by Glassbook.com of Waltham, MA, MightyWords.com of Santa Clara, CA, and Softlock.com of Maynard, MA. Printing and binding by LithoColor Press of Westchester, IL.

Afterwords

End of summer was a transition time. Filling everyone with sorrow, F.K.'s mother died on August 18, 1999. He and I made an attempt to communicate after that, but it fizzled out.

I moved to Michigan that same month and started a nonprofit organization called LocalMotion, dedicated to clarifying the links between environmental toxins and cancer. If there is one reasonable thing we can do about cancer, it is try to eliminate conscious and unconscious poisoning of our own environment.

After a delightful summer in Maine, Ellen returned home and started radiation treatments. By the time they were over, her chest area had taken a beating. Christmas was quiet at the Grayson house, but there was much to celebrate for her treatments were over and she was rebounding.

Ellen kicked off the New Year with exciting vigor. She went to New York for an old friend's birthday party. She traveled to California and spent a few days alone at a desert retreat (a house in Lone Pine) that belonged to a friend. She walked and wrote and loved the high sky. It was a pivotal trip in some ways because it was one of her first ventures out into the world since her diagnosis. She saw her brother and some dear friends and remembered that relationships take work as well as give warmth. A few weeks after that, she went out to Wyoming to see her younger sister. The two of them strapped their babies into colorful sleds and traipsed around the snow-covered hills behind Pam's house.

Sometime in the Fall, Roger became a transformed man by becoming as present with Ellen as he possibly could. When I'd visit, he and Ellen laughed and joked with renewed spirit and happiness. They started marriage counseling in the spring and Ellen was excited and relieved by the way it helped them.

Ellen spent a lot of time preparing for the ritual ceremony she planned to have on her 40th birthday. She finally decided on a church ceremony in which select people would talk about various subjects—love, gratitude, wisdom, sacrifice, hope. Her goal was to show that the good things that had helped her heal were available to us all. Sometime over the birthday weekend, she hoped to bury the breast tissue she had saved from her mastectomy.

In April, Roger and Ellen went to hunt for antiques together in Philadelphia, a weekend event which represents one of their annual rituals. Last year Roger had gone alone; Ellen went to the emergency room. This year things were decidedly and happily different.

In Philadelphia, however, Ellen noticed the waist of a new suit she'd bought for the occasion was uncomfortably tight. When she got home, she visited her internist, who immediately scheduled blood tests and a liver biopsy.

The cancer was back.

Doctors found a tumor on her liver, a spot on her lung, another on a lymph node. She has renewed her struggle.

When she told me the news we cried on the phone with each other. "I'm sorry Betsy, but I'm going to have to drag you back into all of this. Can you research liver metastasis? I'm going to need a lot of survivor stories."

I was finishing up some work in the sunniness of Bermuda and found a cybercafe. I dug in and found that yes, people survive metastasis. One woman had a recurrence in her liver five years ago and is now completely free of the disease. Another woman had her recurrence 13 years ago. The list of survivors is growing. I passed everything on to Ellen and we were both buoyed by the good news. I also sent her a page of treatment options which she took to her oncologist's office. Unfortunately, these treatments won't work for Ellen. She is relying on homeopathic and herbal remedies.

Throughout this long ordeal I have told Ellen about many Internet sites I thought might be of interest to her. She never looked at any of them herself. I was a filter for her. She didn't want to take the risk of reading something that might set off a sense of fear.

"I have to shelter myself from this information," she said. "Whether you get it from the Internet or from a doctor—it's a tremendous psychological danger."

My research gave Ellen context. I could tell her what I'd learned about the treatments, drugs and various other ideas she was interested in. And when doctors told her about something that I'd already read about, it gave the medical advice real-world validation.

When I told her this book was coming along well and nearly done, she asked, "But Betsy, what is the ending going to be?"

VISIT US ONLINE @ FIRSTAIDYOURSELF.ORG

Recommend this Book to a Friend

If you have found *First Aid Yourself* to be a useful and valuable resource please recommend it to your friends. If they want to know more about it immediately, please tell them to see the eBook edition. Recipients do not have to purchase the eBook to sample it; the first 29 pages are open and readable. The entire work may be unlocked, read and stored on computer by completing the simple online transaction form.

Tell your friends to go to the FirstAidYourself Website
(http://www.firstaidyourself.org)
where they may download the sample eBook edition
and explore for themselves.